PRAISE FOR *LIFTING HEAVY THINGS*

"An empowering guide for anyone who wants to experience exercise as an act of self-care, an exploration of strengths, and a practice of self-trust. More than just an introduction to lifting weights, this book shares a new way of relating to your body."

—**Kelly McGonigal**, author of *The Joy of Movement*

"A unique and beautiful book on working with trauma and healing in an embodied way. This advice is both deep and practical, and can be used by anyone interested in a stereotype-breaking story about trauma and how we might heal from it."

—**Ethan Nichtern**, author of *The Road Home: A Contemporary Exploration of the Buddhist Path*

"*Lifting Heavy Things* takes an innovative and timely approach to addressing trauma. This powerful, embodied practice, combined with a gentle and compassionate emotional perspective, is brilliant. This is a book I will use in my practice with clients working to heal trauma."

—**Haven Fyfe Kiernan**, LICSW, psychotherapist and trauma specialist

"I wouldn't be surprised to see a new movement revolution sparked by Laura's genre-bending book. *Lifting Heavy Things* has 'raised the bar' by revealing how movement can be the satisfying basis of healing trauma."

—**Dan Cayer**, Alexander Technique teacher and contributor to *The In-Between* newsletter

LIFTING
HEAVY
THINGS

LIFTING HEAVY THINGS

Healing Trauma
One Rep at a Time

LAURA KHOUDARI

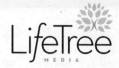

LifeTree
MEDIA

Cataloguing data available from Library and Archives Canada

ISBN 978-1-928055-77-8 (paperback)
ISBN 978-1-928055-78-5 (EPUB)
ISBN 978-1-928055-79-2 (EPDF)

Editor: Jennifer Kurdyla
Copy editor: Sydney Radclyffe
Cover design and interior design: Morgan Krehbiel
Cover image: iStock.com/vav63
Author photo: Viviana Podhaiski

Published by LifeTree Media, an imprint of Wonderwell
www.wonderwell.press

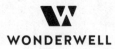

WONDERWELL

Distributed in the US by Publishers Group West and in Canada by Publishers Group Canada

Printed and bound in Canada

CONTENTS

FOREWORD

TRAUMA IS AN UNSPEAKABLY TERRIBLE EXPERIENCE that overwhelms and incapacitates you. It also refers to the resulting underlying and overt feeling of being unsafe that remains in the body and that never completely relaxes. The deep-seated emotional and physiological residue of trauma changes the way you perceive and experience yourself and the world around you. The typical hair-trigger reactions of shutting down, or feeling the urge to flee or fight at the slightest suggestion of danger, become the norm and, in turn, diminish your ability to relate effectively to your world and life.

Traditionally in our Western culture, we have turned to talk therapists to help us make sense of these overwhelming experiences and resolve them. With a good, caring therapist, talking can get you to a place of awareness and acceptance of the events of your life. You may come to understand the reasons you react to triggering situations in certain ways, but understanding is often not enough to help change reactive tendencies or instill the confidence to find new ways of being in the world. In other words, people living with trauma may find that talk therapy alone cannot bring them the relief they are seeking.

For a fuller form of healing from trauma, we need to contend with the physiological states that correspond to our thoughts and emotions. We need to befriend our bodies and learn what is going on internally. This is what is often referred to as embodied awareness. Embodied awareness is not a fixed state that can be achieved once and for all;

it is a fluid and constantly shifting state that requires intention and practice to consistently reestablish as we move through day-to-day life. Paradoxically, embodied awareness can be extremely challenging for people living with trauma to practice, because the feelings of constant threat that trauma instills in the body can make tuning into the body's signals feel intolerably uncomfortable. Therapists who work with embodied awareness–based modalities strive to help their clients return to a sense of safety within their bodies so that lasting healing can take place.

I came to my practices of embodied awareness through personal exploration as a singer-songwriter, a yoga practitioner, a peer counselor; through meditation; through my thirty years of attuned awareness as a massage therapist; and through actor training in theater. Since 2012, I have been guiding embodied awareness experiences in the context of trauma workshops with Bessel van der Kolk, author of the esteemed book on trauma, *The Body Keeps the Score*. I met Laura Khoudari a few years ago at one such workshop I was coleading at Kripalu Center for Yoga & Health in Massachusetts. She was a bright light in a room full of caring people from all walks of life, interested in learning about the role the body plays in the healing of trauma.

After the workshop, we connected on social media. Laura's posts filled me with awe and admiration. Here was this gentle and insightful weight-lifting woman, respectfully encouraging us all to become stronger inside and accept ourselves in the bodies we have.

I always thought that Laura's inspiring words would make a wonderful book, and this book is much more than I imagined or expected. In *Lifting Heavy Things*, Laura shares her techniques for reinhabiting the body through mindful movement and carefully guides us on a journey of self-exploration and courage, providing a step-by-step process of learning how to listen to and trust the self. Her writing voice is that of a warm, confident friend helping you to feel at home in the gym—a place that may not seem so friendly at first to some of us—and anywhere else you might choose to exercise. She generously shares her own journey to strength, as well as the techniques she uses with her clients. Then, always gently and respectfully, she invites you to embark upon your own healing journey through writing prompts, physical exercises, sensory observations, and internal reflections.

This book is a steady, worthy companion for anyone interested in undertaking embodied healing work. May it help you find your way to self-compassion, self-acceptance, a sense of strength, and an embodied awareness practice that can serve you for a lifetime.

—Licia Sky, cofounder of the Trauma Research Foundation

MY TRAUMA STORY
THAT I NEVER TELL

[   ]

AUTHOR'S NOTE
ON PRIVACY

W HEN I TALK ABOUT MY WORK, I invariably mention that
my interest in trauma-informed movement grew out of my
own experience healing from PTSD following an acute trauma in 2014.
People then often ask me, "Can I ask what happened?"

I reply, "No. I'm sorry." My refusal is rarely challenged, and I feel my
body relax with relief.

People ask this for different reasons: some because they care, others
because they cannot help themselves. We all love a good story, and it's
often thought that a good story needs shocking events to keep an audience in its thrall. I disagree. I think a good story is character-driven
and can be interesting without anything terribly exciting happening.
(I hope you think so too, because I've written a book full of stories like
this for you.)

People also share their trauma stories for different reasons, whether
asked or not, but it has been my experience that people often don't
realize they don't have to share. They might believe that, in order to ask
for help or to be of help, they need to explain the details of what they
went through. Again, I disagree—in principle and from experience. I
believe we can receive and give help without telling our trauma story, or
any other part of our story for that matter. Although trauma researchers
and practitioners agree that when healing we need people with whom

to process our trauma story and confide in (both can happen with the same person), we don't have to share everything with *everyone*. We need not prove ourselves to be worthy of help. We do not owe anyone an explanation. And if someone continually asks for details and ignores your boundaries, it's fairly certain they are not a safe person. As such, throughout this book I will use the following marks when I feel the need to bring up the context of my own trauma story: [   ]. Throughout the book, we will explore the healing quality of space, as represented typographically by these brackets and in the form of compassionate pauses—an allowance to go slow or even stop.

To that end, I want to address the way I incorporate my clients' stories in this book. I do so sparingly and have changed their details and blended their stories. I never share a personal trauma narrative (besides, I rarely even know it).

Lastly, I want to note that I began writing this book before the COVID-19 pandemic. At the time, I was thinking deeply about how to convey that we all experience a variety of potential traumas: we lose someone we love; we are involved in accidents or get sick; we are victims of violence or social injustice. But as I neared finishing my first draft, I found myself writing about trauma in the midst of a society-wide trauma, the intensity of which many of us had never experienced before.

Trauma, at a base level, leaves us feeling disempowered, lonely, and fearful. COVID-19 has certainly done this for many folks by instilling fears of loss: the loss of jobs and economic stability, of a known way of life, and of life itself. Everyone is impacted in some way and to some degree. Although this book was not written specifically for life during a pandemic, that context has shaped how I talk in the text about trauma on a macro-level and about accessibility to physical training modalities.

In my own journey and professional studies, I have learned that trauma is the unprocessed physiological response to an overwhelming event or events. Trauma is *not* the narrative of what happened, but a result of the fact that whatever happened was too much or too quick for your nervous system to process in the moment. In turn, the trauma prevents you from moving through and completing your natural threat response cycle, leaving you effectively stuck somewhere in that response even after the threat is gone. Your nervous system may still try to protect you from a threat that is no longer there. This leads to changes in your emotional and physical state that are likely dissonant with the present reality. As a trauma practitioner who works with the body, I have come to understand deep in my own viscera that we can help ourselves and others without focusing on the details of the narrative, but on the feelings, sensations, behavior, images, and meaning left behind. Whether you are working with an acute trauma, like assault or an accident, complex childhood trauma, generational trauma, or a larger societal trauma, it is my intention to help you learn how to tolerate the stress and discomfort it brings, no matter the narrative.

We can hold space for others and ask to be held ourselves without sharing our trauma stories. This book is, in part, an ode to feeling safe in our bodies and in the world. It is also a rallying cry for us to respect one another's humanity, agency, dignity, and privacy. In my work, I can help people without knowing their story—their body tells me all I need to know to guide them on their path to healing. You deserve that space. We all do.

INTRODUCTION

WHEN I WORK WITH CLIENTS INDIVIDUALLY, I understand and appreciate that they are making the choice to include me on their path. The same goes for you, dear reader. Experiencing your own agency is an important piece of trauma work, and I want to acknowledge that you are doing so in choosing to pick up this book. Thank you for including me as a guide on your healing journey.

What I also do when I start working with a client is introduce myself. As such, before we get started, I want to give you the opportunity to learn a bit about me as a practitioner as well as what to expect from this book.

MY EMBODIMENT JOURNEY

I am not your typical fitness professional. I became a trainer and intern at a barbell club in my late thirties. I decided to start my new career path because I felt called to become the trainer I had sought myself, but could not find, following [   ]. I wanted a personal trainer who understood how trauma changes the way people experience their bodies and the world around them. It was my experience, which I later found was supported by research, that exercise had the power to help me heal, but could also exacerbate trauma symptoms.

Immediately following [   ] and before I started doing research, I longed to find a trainer or coach who understood this too and reflected back to me that they also understood what it was like to live with trauma—how hard it was to move well as I struggled to tolerate daily life in my body. As alone as I felt at times, I found it hard to believe that I was the only person out there like me; I wanted to strength train, but trauma was making it difficult for me to feel safe while doing so. I found that without safety, healing was impossible.

And I was right. As soon as I began practicing as a trauma-informed personal trainer, clients around the globe reached out wanting to work using this approach. Over four years I have done some great work with individuals in person, but I want to be able to share the body-based modalities for healing trauma with more folks than I could humanly work with one-on-one. So I wrote this book.

Another thing that makes me different from many fitness professionals is that I am not a jock and never was. Growing up, I hated gym class and was confused by my friends who chose to play sports. Not immediately revealing myself to be coordinated or athletic, my gym teachers and classmates wrote me off as such. I thought I didn't really mind because I was happiest when I was sitting and reading, writing, drawing, or talking to friends (which matched the rest of the rebel persona I had adopted anyhow). But some part of me internalized the idea that I was unathletic and had no business in the gym. I interpreted that to mean my body was less deserving of love than those of my more athletic-appearing peers. Over time, this poor self-esteem around my body, in both its appearance and ability, made me increasingly disinterested in physical activity.

Flash forward twenty years and I have become a fitness professional, my accomplishments even highlighted by my college's alumnae association. The college (where, as a student, I had deigned to participate in mandatory PE for what I thought was the last time in my life) interviewed me for two publications and included a photo of me seated comfortably in workout clothes on a weight bench, a rack of dumbbells in soft focus in the background. Those photos revealed just how much had changed since I graduated. My hair still hangs in curls around my face, but they are no longer dyed purple. My body, still soft and average appearing, is considerably stronger than it was at twenty-two. The most important change is not visible: I understand that my body is mine, that I am entitled to have boundaries around it and to take up space with it.

Next to my photo is a pull quote from the interview: *I came into my voice. And not only did I learn what I wanted to say, I felt ok saying it.* I was referring to my experience of gaining confidence at a women's college as an insecure teen, but these words also apply to my post-graduate experience: through strength training, as an adult woman, and as a trauma survivor. I went from resenting physical activity to doing it begrudgingly, then habitually, and eventually joyfully, over the course of fourteen years. Strength training helps me continue to step further into my power each day, including in writing this book.

The seeds of my own movement practice were planted back in 1999 when my back went out for the first time. It was the summer between my junior and senior years of college, and I was getting out of a chair at my student job when my back seized up all of a sudden. I could barely walk and spent the rest of the summer recuperating so I could be well enough to sit without excruciating pain in long seminars and lectures the next fall. The orthopedist I saw suggested that strength training could alleviate the pain. While I was relieved that he wasn't suggesting surgery, exercise felt punitive because going to the gym was all tied up in a messy knot with my experiences in physical education class in school, my poor self-esteem, and an internalized societal rejection of the shape and size of my body. I did the prescribed physical therapy and then promptly put strength training, and my body, on the back burner.

Three days a week at a local commercial gym, I saw my physical therapist, a reticent young woman with a shaved head dressed in the unofficial physical therapist uniform of a polo and khakis. On arrival I would get on the elliptical for five minutes or so and then we would head into the treatment room, where she'd spend thirty minutes doing soft tissue work on my back and adjacent muscles, relaxing their spasms enough so I could move. She often did this by finding a tender point with her thumb, knuckle, or elbow, and staying with it until it released. Then she would massage the surrounding area and move on to the next tender spot and the next. Then we'd do a few core-strengthening exercises before going back to the elliptical for five minutes. It would be ten minutes the following week, and so on until I could tolerate thirty minutes.

After six weeks of physical therapy I returned to campus with a bit of a limp, a crush on my PT, and the intention of sticking with using the elliptical machine two or three times a week. The limp lasted for years, the crush for days, and my commitment to the gym not at all. I rarely used the elliptical in college. I would only go to the fitness center if nothing else worked for a flare-up of pain and to keep up the habit just until the pain stopped.

Seven long years later, I showed up at New York Sports Club to begin strength training. In the time since that bout of physical therapy, I lived my life by moving around carefully; I was only twenty-seven, but I was frequently in pain and always afraid of my back going out again. I had discovered yoga as one modality that helped reduce my pain levels and cultivated a regular practice, but I still couldn't be pain-free for more than five days. I finally accepted that I wasn't adequately managing my back pain and that my original doctor (not to mention my mom, who was urging me to meet her trainer) was probably right.

The day I showed up to my mom's gym, despite resisting it with every fiber of my being, turned out to be the start of a sustainable and healing movement practice. My first trainer, "Big Ed" Williams, who would become a mentor and lifelong friend, greeted me with a warm and genuine smile. (You'll get to know him better in this book.) Over the course of eight years, Ed would not only help me train to get out of pain; he would create space for me to find pride in my body, as well as have fun in the gym. By our last year of working together, I had also found the curiosity and courage necessary to try the competitive sport of weightlifting (also known as "Olympic weightlifting" or "Olympic lifting," presumably to differentiate it from the act of lifting weights to strength train). You may be familiar with the event from the summer Olympics, in which athletes use three lifts to get barbells weighing hundreds of pounds off the ground and up over their heads.

It took a couple more years before my movement practice evolved into its current form: embodied, healing, and joyful. Following [   ] I developed PTSD, and then sustained a second back injury that left me unable to do much of anything, especially Olympic lifting. In order to feel safe training, I decided to use movement to intentionally cultivate a relationship with my body; I listened to it more carefully and began to honor it, not just when it needed to move but also when it needed to rest. I had to, or else I ran the risk of getting hurt again and again, which would mean I couldn't train at all. I changed the way I approached strength training in order to heal my back first, then to protect my body. I had no idea that this mental process would also play a pivotal role in helping me heal my emotional and spiritual self, as well as my relationships with others.

DISCOVERING EMBODIED PRACTICE

I deepened my practice, while also achieving long-term training goals, through self-directed education and practical exploration. I sought out classes and studied with trauma teachers and practitioners who worked with the physiology of trauma. It was during my initial studies that I decided to become a certified personal trainer, so I cracked those books, too—my shelves now bend under the weight of the books I have read on the physiology of trauma, Somatic Experiencing, mindfulness practices, polyvagal theory and its application to healing trauma, trauma-sensitive yoga, and human movement. These are the various modalities I use myself and with clients, some of which we'll get into in this book.

In books and through experience, I've learned that our bodies have a lot of good information to share if we pay attention. This happens when we're in a state commonly referred to as "embodied," which is thrown around a lot in wellness circles without a very clear definition. We're all in bodies, right? So how can we not be embodied? Unfortunately, that's not quite everything.

When you are embodied, you are mindful of your body—its shape, weight, and density—and have the capacity to be aware of feelings and sensations that arise from it as and when they do (not after or before). It may sound simple to be embodied, but for many people it's not—especially those living with trauma (we'll go into this in Part II).

I first figured out how to be embodied in the gym and then in the world. This process helped me discover what I was capable of and what my boundaries, needs, joys and fears are. I stumbled a lot along the way. I spent a lot of money and time on orthopedists and physical therapists, body workers and energy workers, hypnotherapists and talk therapists, mindfulness and yoga classes, personal trainers and weight-lifting coaches, wellness retreats and workshops, feng shui experts, and of course, books on all of these subjects! Of the many therapeutic modalities I tried, some worked for me and others didn't.

By teaching you in this book how to listen to what your whole body tells you, I hope to help you bypass the services, modalities, and practitioners out there that don't align with what you want and need from your own long-term journey with healing through movement. From an embodied place, you will be better equipped to decide what is actually safe and healing for you, as opposed to doing things because others tell you they're safe and healing. Although my story is one that takes place primarily in the weight room, I know that yours may take place elsewhere—a Pilates studio, your own living room, or the great outdoors, to name a few places where embodiment may await you. The tools I share in these pages will work, no matter which movement sparks your curiosity and no matter where you practice.

ABOUT ME

I think it's important for you as my reader to learn more about me generally along with the parts of my daily experience that have shaped my work, because these formed the lens I bring to my work and my writing. My work grew out of all of my own lived experiences, and my healing and growing was shaped by many factors that go beyond my trauma. My experience has roots in areas where I have had tremendous privilege, such as wealth and perceived whiteness and heterosexuality, which gave me access to a private education from high school through graduate school and have opened doors to networks of people who could help me. My privilege has also granted me access to excellent medical and mental healthcare, as well as making it possible for me to access many different wellness modalities.

My experience is also that of a Jewish American of Syrian descent who is not always seen as white. While I have benefitted from white supremacy, I have also experienced racism. I am queer and often assumed to be heterosexual because I married a cisgender man. I have experienced heterosexism. And like my sexuality, they may not be visible, but I am living with disabilities. I have experienced ableism.

I am also about a size twelve or fourteen. I have an average appearing physique. I mention this because although people come in all shapes and sizes, a lot of folks feel movement is off-limits to them, not because of ability but simply because they are not lean or small. I live in a body that is larger and softer than most fitness professionals', yet I work in the fitness space. I have been told by colleagues I don't belong because I am "unhealthy." They don't actually mean unhealthy—it is code for fat. In terms of my health, my bloodwork is excellent. I have healthy relationships, a fulfilling life, and a strong sense of my own boundaries. Those people, however, suffer from fatphobia. I have experienced body shame.

Professionally, I have worked with clients in barbell clubs, personal trainer facilities, and remotely with clients in their own homes or gyms. In barbell clubs, my clientele was diverse in age, gender, race and sexuality. My private clients tend to be white, cisgender women or gender non-conforming people in their late-twenties and thirties.

WHY STRENGTH TRAINING?

There are many movement-based modalities and more are being invented every day. For some of us, our movements can appear to flow one into the next, whereas others move more abruptly or forcefully. Some of us may move more stiffly and others appear floppy. But at the end of the day, our skeletons are designed to move in a finite number of ways; our joints hinge and sometimes swivel, our muscles contract and relax, and our nervous systems make it all happen. Human movement in all its forms comes from the movement systems working together: muscles, bones, and nerves all communicating in the same language.

This really sunk in for me one day when I was in a yoga class practicing the pose Warrior III. About two years ago, after countless times doing the pose where you stand on one leg, lift the other leg behind you, and lean your upper body forward to make a T shape, I realized it's the same movement as a single-leg Romanian deadlift—something I'd done at the gym to improve performance. They are both hip hinges done on one leg. The only difference is the *assumed* approach to them. It is assumed in yoga that one is moving mindfully through the shapes, uniting breath with movement and maintaining presence of mind. That said, I know many people (past me included) who spend yoga class focusing on perception and performance—how to look the best, or even "win" doing yoga.

On the flip side, many folks assume strength training is all about performance and appearance. I am going to be honest with you: my unyielding desire to look like a strong badass is what got me under the barbell in the first place and is part of my motivation to keep coming back. But when I train now, it's no longer a performance or in the name of performance. I don't train to compete in weightlifting anymore and I don't expect to win anything when I'm done with a session. That mentality doesn't align with my own goals for training anymore.

I train to feel my body, uniting my breath to reps and focusing on what it feels like inside as my body moves against the resistance of the weight of kettlebells, dumbbells, barbells and more. In that way, I approach strength training the way one is intended to approach yoga. I train to deepen my relationship with myself and to feel my capacity for lifting heavy things. I train to be embodied.

Along with all of this awesome stuff, strength training—lifting weights, using weight machines, and training with resistance bands— benefits your heart, muscles, bones, posture, and balance. It makes you a more efficient mover and can eliminate certain types of chronic pain. It improves your mood and promotes better sleep. On top of all of these benefits, the experience of getting physically stronger over time builds feelings of self-confidence and self-efficacy, which is very empowering. While some of my clients have worked with me to become powerlifters, most of them are focused on everyday empowerment: being able to carry their groceries home, take long bike rides with their partners, or feel confident enough to take a group fitness class.

In terms of working with trauma, I find embodied strength training incredibly useful in cultivating a sense of safety within one's own body, as well as helping survivors identify what they need to feel safe in their environment and relationships. In her seminal book *Trauma and Recovery: The Aftermath of Violence—from Domestic Abuse to Political Terror*, Dr. Judith Herman, a professor of psychiatry at Harvard Medical School, proposed a three-stage model for recovery from psychological trauma. The first stage is establishing a sense of safety, starting from within the body and then moving outward into the environment. She recommends "hard exercise" as one method to manage stress and promote a feeling of safety in the body.[1] She does not define "hard exercise," but I interpret it to mean exercise that gets your heart pumping and activates your central nervous system. Depending on how you approach your workout, this can be done with resistance equipment to increase strength. More generally, she notes that any exercise gives survivors the opportunity to tend to their own body in a way that promotes a sense of autonomy. Herman also mentions that the first stage is a good place to address issues around interrupted sleep, insomnia being a common trauma symptom. Exercise that builds muscle like strength training has been found to be associated with better sleep.[2]

No modality works for everybody all of the time, but sometimes it feels like it should—in the case of trauma survivors, we might feel like yoga is supposed to work for us. Many trauma survivors, myself included, find yoga (even the trauma-informed kind) quite triggering. I note this because, although trauma-informed trainers, coaches and teachers in most modalities are scarce, you are likely to be able to find trauma-informed yoga instruction if you live near a major metropolitan area. While trauma-informed yoga is relatively available, it isn't for everyone, and it can be disheartening (even devastating) if it doesn't work for you and you think it's the only form of exercise available to you as a trauma survivor. This was my own experience. I tried to return to yoga following [   ] and, though I previously had a regular practice for ten years, it felt like a physical and emotional minefield. On the other hand, I was triggered far less often by strength training and was able to bounce back from upsetting moments in the gym more quickly than from those on the yoga mat. You might find strength training to be supportive too, but you might also find another modality altogether as your sweet spot for embodiment.

That said, I firmly believe that any modality can be practiced in a trauma-sensitive way, and that people who are recovering from trauma would benefit from more information and options for trauma-informed movement practices. In a 2018 study of women survivors of sexual violence, most participants felt that engaging in exercise, whether it was high intensity (elevating the heart rate) or low-impact (like yoga), came with the risk of being triggered, especially in the early stages of recovery. At the same time, all participants also felt exercise was beneficial to their healing path.[3]

The truth is that when living with trauma, you run the risk of being triggered by all sorts of stimuli—even in environments designed to be therapeutic. As such, the questions to ask yourself if you want to start using movement in your healing work are: 1) What modality is least likely to feel triggering for me? and 2) How can I quickly recover from triggering moments? This book is partly intended to help you answer both questions for yourself, even if you don't choose strength training or don't do it exclusively.

WHY THIS BOOK IS FOR YOU

I have written this book primarily for anyone living with trauma who is curious about incorporating movement or exercise into their healing path, and I am writing to you as I would speak to a client. Therapists, personal trainers, and other fitness professionals may also find this book useful as a model of how to use exercise to complement other healing practices.

When it comes to trauma, although we all have unique and different experiences, trauma symptoms impact the body in much the same way from one person to another. Clients come to me with post-traumatic stress disorder, postpartum depression, postpartum anxiety, fibromyalgia, chronic fatigue syndrome, depression, and anxiety. Clients have also come to me with experiences of addiction, eating disorders, and other conditions. While I'm not a specialist in any of these fields, lifting heavy things can provide support to people healing from trauma and mitigating its impact on their lives. The tools provided here are intended to be used by anyone as a complement to their healing process. However, working with me or with this book isn't a substitute for professional mental health or medical advice, diagnosis, or treatment.

I have tried to be inclusive in writing this book, giving consideration to issues around access and privilege. I remain committed to learning the ways in which my privilege has led to blind spots in my teaching while I continue to show up in hope of facilitating social change through my trauma work. I am a firm believer that no coach is for everybody, including me, but it is also my hope that many people with their own varied stories, backgrounds, and experiences feel seen, heard, and helped by this book.

HOW TO TRAIN WITH THIS BOOK

This book is broken into three sections: Conditions, Activation, and Recovery. This three-part structure mimics the flow of a workout I might design for a client or use myself.

In Part I, I explain how to establish what you'll need to create a trauma-healing movement practice. Before you begin a workout, you probably put on exercise clothes, gather necessary equipment and supplies (water bottle, yoga mat, etc.) and maybe head to a specific location. You are putting the conditions in place to exercise. In this section, you'll meet my favorite weightlifting coach, Coach Kenny, as well as the aforementioned

"Big Ed" Williams and a childhood bully of mine. Each of them, for better or for worse, helped me identify what I needed to put in place in order to feel okay before setting foot in the gym and training. We'll look at how trauma impacts your nervous system and your tolerance for exercise, and we'll explore shifting your mindset around exercise and giving you the tools to feel prepared and safe while you move.

Next, you'll get to it and get active! Part II is about turning a movement practice into an embodied one. We'll see how a regular practice of embodied movement while engaging in exercise can help you "feel into" your agency, and identify and enforce your boundaries. These skills are crucial to feeling safe enough to engage in healing work. In Part II you will read some client stories, hear from an expert in a trauma-healing modality called Somatic Experiencing, and meet a well-intentioned but pushy friend of mine. We'll explore the ways trauma inhibits us from being fully present in our bodies, then delve into what an embodied movement practice is and the practicalities of creating one. We'll also look at how the empowering benefits of this practice can radiate to other areas of your life as well.

Lastly, you'll cool down—stretch, drink some water, and hopefully pat yourself on the back for taking the time to tend to yourself. You are setting yourself up for recovery. Part III goes into what life during recovery looks like once you have experienced embodiment, as you learn to connect with and listen to your body. In a workout, recovery happens after the session, but the healing journey is less compartmentalized and linear; as you learn to connect with yourself in Parts I and II, you may find yourself laying the groundwork for what is presented in Part III. I'll introduce you to my grandmother Gloria, a 1982-era Jane Fonda, a counseling psychologist with a background in sports psychology and a passion for fitness, and David, my partner and true love. We'll talk about recovery from a fitness perspective: the role of the cool down at the end of a movement session and how recovery from the stress of exercise helps build nervous system resilience. More broadly, recovery includes finding the right movement practice for you—one that is sustainable and, hopefully, joyful—as well as learning how to incorporate other people in your healing, potentially sharing your story, and knowing what to do when you feel stuck.

At the end of each chapter, you'll see a section called "Take Action." This is a space for interactive exercises; some are related to working out or are writing-based, and some are about relying on the senses. These practical learning tools are intended to help you build an embodied movement practice that suits you and are by no means obligatory. I invite you to try these on your own schedule, whether that's as you read the book or by coming back to them later. I do suggest that you read each one all the way through before starting it. Each exercise begins with a brief explanation of why I chose it, a list of what you will need to do the exercise, and the approximate amount of time it will take. The materials needed vary but are minimal.

While the suggestions and Take Action activities are designed to be accessible to beginners and experts alike, you get to decide if something is or isn't for you. And you get to change your mind. Please listen to your body and don't do anything that hurts or feels "too" anything—too hard, too slow, too fast, too stimulating, too boring. When something is "too" much of anything, there's a risk of feeling overwhelmed. If you find this to be the case, please don't hesitate to find support that feels right to you. This might be a movement coach, trainer, counselor, or another person with whom you do healing work.

And as always, check with a medical professional to see if any of the movements are contraindicated for you.

Like in a well-designed workout, the order of movements matters, and although I suggest that you make your way through this book as it is laid out, you don't have to. You can use this book however you want. Literally. Use it as a hand weight, or as a balance tool, or even as a coaster; but I think you'll get the most out of it if you read it in order, all the way to the end. You can always refer back to past chapters later, as the information and exercises do build on one another. That said, you may find it more useful to skip around according to your own healing journey and your experience with body-based healing practices, and you have the right to do so.

Each of you brings your own experiences to your reading of this book and each of you is at a different point along your healing path, so as you choose how much to read at a given time and at what pace, I want to remind you of something that is at the heart of healing from trauma: you are the expert in you. You are free to pause as often and for as long as you like, or to skip things entirely. This experience is yours. And while I am here as a guide, you are choosing this journey and you can choose to let me join you for a bit or not.

To that end, every time you are about to read, I invite you to take a moment to check in with yourself and pay attention to how you feel. Notice your surroundings: what do you see and hear? Ask yourself if where you are seated feels good. If not, I invite you to take a moment to adjust. Perhaps add a pillow behind your back or turn on a reading lamp, or get up and move to a completely different place. Take a minute to tend to your physical comfort as best you can.

As you read, I will invite you to pause—literally. Throughout the book, you will be prompted in writing to pause and take a moment to check in, and then to engage in a small act of self-care. This is something I do with both clients and myself after some heavy lifting. Please also feel free to pause even when I haven't prompted you. Check in with yourself and notice whether the words are sinking in and making sense or might as well be gibberish. If the concepts aren't sinking in, pause your reading. Maybe stretch or get a glass of water. Look around the room and listen. Ask yourself if you would like to keep reading. There are natural breaks in the book, but you may need pauses in different places to really take in and process what you are reading. That's okay. You picked up this book for you, so approach it at the speed that best serves you.

This book is also intended to be a point of connection between you and the larger world. With it, I hope to make the space necessary for folks living with trauma disorders to feel seen and have their realities recognized. Because at the root of it, trauma is a deeply isolating experience, yet it demands connection in order to heal. Although I had supportive, caring loved ones to help me with [   ], they couldn't understand that my experience of them and of the whole world around me had since changed. I was different. Because I couldn't seem to convey my experience, I was alone in it and felt deeply misunderstood.

Then I started reading about the brain science of trauma, and the words on the page began to normalize the uncontrollable and confusing shifts I felt in myself. This foundation gave me hope that I could heal from what I'd feared was a permanent change. Writing this book has given me the opportunity to do the same for you, in my own voice, with the trauma-sensitive approach I take to lifting heavy things—both literally and figuratively. The process of writing was healing in itself because it asked me to pause, slow down and reflect on the path I've taken, and on the hard work that goes into healing. In those moments, I had the opportunity to appreciate the magnitude of what I have achieved. Healing is hard work and it's nice to really recognize that for myself, as I also recognize it for you.

When I part ways with my clients, I give them the tools to help their transition into the next stage of practicing movement with ease. So at the end of this book, I have done the same for you by including an annotated list of resources for further study. This list is by no means comprehensive as the field of trauma studies is rapidly growing, but it reflects the jumping off point for my own study and work. I now offer it as an entry point for you to deepen your own practice and continue to heal beyond our time together.

TAKE ACTION
Conduct Your Own Intake

Before I start training with a client, I conduct an intake, which serves a number of purposes. It allows me to understand their goals and identify any conditions they need to meet in order to train, as well as the resources, people, places and things that support them. Once I have this sort of information, I come up with a training program and recovery plan tailored to their goals, needs, and lifestyle.

In this exercise I'm inviting you to conduct your own intake, so that as you move forward with your own training program, with the guidance of this book and beyond, you'll know what conditions you need in place, what your resources are, and what your goals are.

WHAT YOU WILL NEED:
2-3 pieces of paper to write lists on
A writing instrument
A timer (optional)

DURATION:
About 20 to 30 minutes

1. IDENTIFY YOUR THREE MAIN REASONS FOR TRAINING

Take a blank piece of paper, set a timer for three minutes, and write down all of the reasons that you are considering training.

- Write down anything that comes to mind and don't censor yourself.
- After three minutes, circle the first three things that feel achievable or that you think you could make measurable progress in over the next three months. Don't think too much about it—just circle what jumps out at you. Acknowledging why you want to make a change in your life is not easy and being guided by your intuition can make that process feel more accessible and realistic.

Tuck this list away, put it on your fridge, or write it on your bathroom vanity with a dry-erase marker. You will refer to it again.

2. IDENTIFY THE CONDITIONS YOU NEED TO TRAIN

Set a timer for five minutes and, on a piece of paper, brainstorm the conditions you need in place to begin to train. Here are some things to consider:

- What are some of your environmental needs? This may include the type of facility, distance from your home, amount of space, and general equipment you'll need to pursue your goals, including clothing, footwear, and music.
- Do you need a formal training program, coaching, or group support?
- At what time of day would you need to train? Consider mealtimes.
- Do you require changing rooms or showers?
- Do you require gender neutral changing rooms or showers?
- Do you require elevators or ramps if the facility is not at street level?
- Do you require that the space upholds an explicit commitment to inclusivity?

After five minutes, review your list and circle anything that is a must-have as opposed to a would-like-to-have. That said, it is okay to circle everything on your list!

3. CREATE A PLAN TO PUT THOSE CONDITIONS IN PLACE

Now consider things you already have that will support your needs. For example:

- A gym membership and access to the gym
- Resistance bands, dumbbells, or other small equipment—even odd objects like books and backpacks and water jugs at home (see Chapter Four for more on setting up a home practice)
- A favorite playlist and some headphones

Put a check mark next to each condition that you can put in place now, without taking action. Now circle what you still need to figure out. For these remaining items you may have to do research or save some money, or you may just need to buy them. Make a plan to put these conditions in place that has concrete steps and action dates.

4. IDENTIFY YOUR RESOURCES

Next you are going to identify resources (people and things that support you in your life) that you can call upon as you pursue your goals. I invite you to answer the following questions:

- What hobbies or activities do you enjoy doing?
- Who supports you in your life?
- Do you have any pets? If so, name them.
- Did you ever play a sport? If so, which sport?
- Do you like to dance? If yes, which kind of dance? (Including random dance parties at home!)
- What's your favorite kind of music?
- Do you have a spiritual practice?
- Are you a member/volunteer of any club or organization?
- Do you have someone from whom you obtain regular counseling?
- Do you have any tokens or talismans with special meaning to you?

Review your lists. I suggest you keep them together and someplace close at hand, so as you go forward you can check in on reasons, needs, and be reminded of your resources.

PART I
CONDITIONS

Before you lift heavy things, you
need to put a few conditions in
place for the work to be fruitful.

CHAPTER ONE

Preparing to Lift Heavy Things

"**C**ONDITIONS FIRST," Coach Kenny reminds me. His voice, relatively quiet, cuts through the cacophony of dance music, loaded barbells crashing down on the platform, and young athletes yelling over everything. It is a weeknight around 5:00 p.m. at JDI Barbell, and it's busy, crowded, and hot. Although small, the gym has two sides: one for the sport of powerlifting (a barbell sport that consists of testing maximal weight that can be lifted in the squat, bench, and deadlift), and one for the sport of weightlifting, which is the side where I am at the moment. I'm sharing the platform with two other women, and the coach is working with six of us at once. I am crouched above a barbell, my hands covered in chalk, positioned far from each other in a wide grip. My body shifts slightly as I create more tension across my back and down into my arms. My chest and gaze rise, and I lift my hips slightly to feel tension ripple down the back of my legs as they adjust into start position.

I take in a breath, simultaneously bracing for the lift and all the distractions surrounding me. I can feel that some folks are watching me and there is a little extra pressure because, when I stand on the powerlifting side of the gym, I am a coach. Fortunately, weightlifting is a really hard sport so no one expects me to be any good at it.

I push the floor away, attempting to move slowly at first and accelerating as the bar passes my knees, with the intention of exploding at the very top of the pull. As the bar moves up it swings forward slightly, creating an arc on its way up overhead instead of moving straight up. I drop down under the bar to catch it overhead in a squat, then stand upright with it. I appear to move fast under the bar, but I know I only looked fast because I cut corners. I did not fully extend my hips as I should have. I exploded both too soon and not enough. With the bar overhead, I shake my head and look at Kenny, then control the descent of the bar until it's just inches away from the floor before releasing it with a dull reverb and a small bounce. He knows that I know everything I did wrong.

He nods. "Again. Conditions first."

In this case, the conditions Kenny is referring to are: keeping my weight in my midfoot so I can push myself straight up; keeping the muscles of my upper back engaged so I can pull the bar up rather than swinging it out; bracing my trunk to protect my back and to create a connection between my upper and lower limbs; and staying focused on the task at hand and not the thousands of other stimuli buzzing around me. *Sure, no problem, Kenny*, I think.

On my second attempt, I do a much better job. The bar moves along a straighter path and I catch it and stand up with it again. But I still don't fully extend. This lack of extension is a habit that I am working to correct. My body does it to protect me, and although it works with lighter weights it does not serve me as the weight increases toward the maximum amount I can hold over my head.

I like practicing lifting heavy things. There is a ritual around showing up, gearing up, setting up, and drilling with a focus on the technical minutiae of a lift in the name of being able to stand up with more and more weight. And I like practicing with Kenny in particular. Not all barbell clubs or coaches have felt right for me. I'm particular, but I feel safe being coached by Kenny at JDI. His coaching style resonates with me. Sometimes we talk about work, food, or training when it's quiet in the gym and I am between sets. He is approachable and kind but not particularly chatty or ebullient while coaching. His steady presence is nice in an environment filled with explosive energy. He almost never yells, not even over the other sounds just to be heard. He says "do it again" a lot, occasionally expanding with, "add weight." That means I'm doing a good job. He holds the space simply by showing up and making sure that the chaos on the platforms around his clients is not coming into their space, too.

Prior to [   ], I had been training to lift some pretty heavy things: I could squat with weights upward of 175 pounds for 10 reps and was progressing steadily, gaining strength over time. But after [   ], my progress halted and even moderately intense training was a struggle. I couldn't tolerate the feeling of that much weight bearing down on me. I hadn't yet processed [   ] and I didn't feel safe in the gym—or even in my body—and I didn't understand why. I wasn't at JDI when [   ] happened, although I doubt it would have made much difference, because the issue was one that was inside of me, not around me. For the first few months, I would experience flashbacks in the squat rack, even though my trauma had nothing to do with the gym. The physical stress of exercise was too great for me to tolerate—I was already walking around in a state of chronic activation—and heavy weight on my back made me feel trapped and triggered terror. Bar on my back, body quaking, stuck and frozen, I would try to fend off intrusive thoughts and memories. But there was no escaping them as they flashed before my eyes, which darted around in their sockets looking for something else to land on. A fog would sometimes creep in as if through my ear canal, across my brain, and over my eyes.

"No!" I would yell, grunt, or grunt-whimper at my fatigue and frustration, and I would rerack the bar, sometimes without doing a single rep. "I don't want to lose this, too," I would think. The "too" referred to the sense of control and safety I had lost in every other sphere of my life. Turning on the television, picking up my daughter at school, or going into the office all felt like I was about to walk into a labyrinth with the risk of peril lurking behind each turn. Any feeling of safety in this world was gone, and I didn't know exactly why, but I knew it had to do with [   ].

Determined to train, I kept the weights light as I attempted to clean up my technique on an Olympic lift called the snatch, but I shook so hard between sets that coaches and other athletes would ask me if I was okay. "Yes. I just shake is all. I'm nervous, I guess," I would say, feeling vulnerable, which in turn felt scary, which made me shake more. In hindsight, I can see all the messages my body was sending me to take a pause, but I didn't then. I kept at it, refusing to take a break from the sport, worried that if I stopped it would vanish from my life. I was certain that if I just kept training, the uncontrollable feelings would go away. I was wrong.

*I invite you to pause, check in, and move part
of your body, even just a little bit.*

A SHORT LESSON ON TRAUMA AND THE BRAIN

Before we can lift heavy things—like trauma or barbells—we must put the conditions in place. One of the first conditions for lifting heavy things to heal from trauma is that you have a basic understanding of how trauma impacts your brain and nervous system. It has been my experience that understanding why you suddenly feel weird and unsafe in familiar environments or relationships can empower you to begin to do the hard work of healing. Although it may seem a trite expression, knowledge really is power. It will also help you begin to recognize trauma symptoms for what they are and to address them accordingly.

In my studies as a trauma practitioner, I have learned some basic models of the brain and always share these models when talking to new clients, students, or even other folks who are trying to understand what it is I do. Now I am going to share them with you. It is important that you have a basic understanding of what is happening in your brain and body when you become so overwhelmed you cannot process information, change, and heal.

The brain is complicated. It doesn't just process whatever you're aware you are thinking about; it is also constantly processing what you see, smell, taste, hear, feel, and how you move through your environment. Your brain controls your body's interconnected systems and the way it responds to the world around you. It's also where those thoughts about your experiences, past and present, come from.

The brain can be broken down into a number of parts, but for our purposes let's focus on three: the brain stem, the limbic system, and the neocortex.

Your brain stem controls basic things like eating, sleeping, elimination, and arousal. It also works with parts of your limbic system (and the parts of your brain that deal with higher-order processes) to choose how to mobilize under threat: fight, flight, or freeze. Without it, you wouldn't stay alive very long. It remembers that the stove is hot and produces a response in fractions of a millisecond when you put your hand near the flame, bypassing the much bigger, but slower-processing parts of your brain. This is why you'll often find yourself jumping out of the way of danger before you realize what you are doing on a more conscious level. In addition, your limbic system regulates how you experience and react to emotions, affecting interactions and the relationships you form with others. It helps create memories of events, facts, and feelings. We spend a lot of time with this system in trauma work, because trauma results from an interrupted trauma-induced limbic response.

Next comes the neocortex. We are only concerned with one part of that structure here, which is called the prefrontal cortex. This is the rational part of the brain, concerned with executive functioning. It's where you process abstract thoughts and concepts (like time), make mental connections, and can acknowledge and get perspective on feelings, both your own and others' (which is the root of empathy). It is home to your moral compass, your insight, and your intuition. And it's also where you can quiet your fear through reason.

You need to be in touch with this system to make meaning of your experiences. When you become overwhelmed, the wise prefrontal cortex is not engaged. Instead, your emotional yet tough-as-nails survivalist limbic system becomes wide awake. The limbic system is commonly associated with fight and flight, not thought. When it's in charge, you're unable to make new connections from the information around you. Instead, you are flooded by emotion and rely on memory to draw conclusions, make meaning, and act.

Here's how this might play out. Imagine that you have had a really bad day at work and the commute home was horrific. Maybe you have kids and when you walk in the door, they are acting up, too. You haven't been sleeping well because of work stress, and then a loved one makes a comment you don't like. Imagine that in response, you fly off the handle, only to later realize you overreacted because of everything else going on. It was your limbic system that responded to your loved one, and later your prefrontal cortex came online to create the thought, "Oh, that was wrong. I didn't mean to take my day out on them."

Being embodied requires your prefrontal cortex to be online, so that you can make meaning of the sensations and feelings that arise in your body as you experience them. This might be challenging, or even impossible, if your system is constantly managing stress from unprocessed trauma. When your baseline stress levels are already high, it is easy to become overwhelmed and move into a limbic state—and possibly even stay there.

THE WINDOW OF TOLERANCE

Being unable to regulate the dance between the prefrontal cortex and limbic system presents a few problems when working with trauma, whether using movement or otherwise. With the prefrontal cortex offline, you can neither take care of yourself as you operate in real time, nor integrate any new skills. Your nervous system will be too overwhelmed. When Coach Kenny reminded me, "conditions first," I used my prefrontal cortex to think about what I was doing before I did it. If I couldn't do that because my limbic system was in charge, then I'd be trying to lift a large amount of weight over my head without awareness of how I was moving. I would be more likely to both miss the lift and get hurt. Likewise, if you were in a limbic state during a conversation, like in talk therapy, you would likely get swept up in your feelings rather than processing and integrating them. However, when your prefrontal cortex is online and controlling your responses

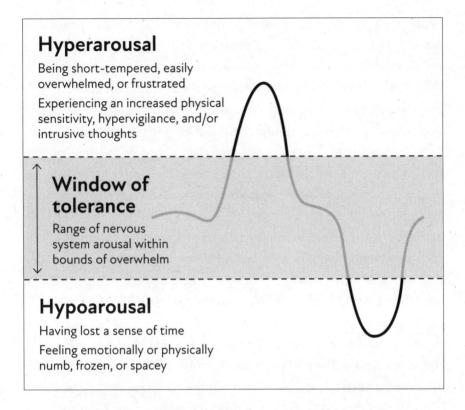

Hyperarousal

Being short-tempered, easily overwhelmed, or frustrated

Experiencing an increased physical sensitivity, hypervigilance, and/or intrusive thoughts

Window of tolerance

Range of nervous system arousal within bounds of overwhelm

Hypoarousal

Having lost a sense of time

Feeling emotionally or physically numb, frozen, or spacey

to whatever is going on, you can keep your cool, think about your thoughts, and learn new things.

Mental health practitioners describe this state as "being in your window of tolerance." Dr. Dan Siegel—an internationally renowned neuropsychiatrist, clinical professor of psychiatry at the UCLA School of Medicine, and executive director of the Mindsight Institute—created this illustrative model in 1999. (He is also a skillful teacher, able to simplify and explain complex scientific concepts for a wide variety of audiences; I recommend his work to anyone who's interested.) The window of tolerance depicts the range of nervous system arousal anyone might experience, from hyperarousal to hypo (a lack of) arousal. The middle of the arousal spectrum—the "window of tolerance" for which the model is named—is where we want to be most of the time. The window is the range of nervous system arousal an individual can tolerate without becoming overwhelmed and either hyper or hypo-aroused. Stressors, both good (like healing work and working out) and bad (like arguments and toilet paper shortages) can still occur when we're within this window, but we are better able to tolerate the discomfort and our responses remain organized.

I like this model, because we can use it to understand that everyone's capacity for stress is different and that being overwhelmed takes many varied forms. Also like a window's opening, tolerance can be further opened or closed. Throughout this book, I will refer to the window of tolerance when talking about stressors and increasing our capacity for them.

A healthy nervous system fluctuates in its response to stimuli. Even on a perfectly boring day with no workouts, arguments, or crises, your arousal levels will fluctuate—when you eat, encounter other people, read the news, and generally go about living your life. This is necessary for your nervous system to do its job, which is to tell the rest of the body how to respond to your environment. However, when you encounter a stimulus that's too much to handle, you either move up into hyperarousal (shown above the window of tolerance) or down into hypoarousal (shown below the window of tolerance). And when you are in either of these states, your limbic system is in the driver's seat, not your prefrontal cortex.

What pushes us over the edge (or out the window) may be something commonly deemed traumatic, such as experiencing or witnessing violence, being in an accident, or losing a loved one. But if you are already under a lot of stress—grappling with the realities of racism, homophobia, misogyny, ableism, fatphobia, or ageism; living with abuse; navigating life during a pandemic; or going through a painful divorce, among other things—or if your window of tolerance is narrow for any other reason, then a sudden loud noise, an argument with a loved one, or a near accident may be enough to overwhelm you.

When you are hyperaroused, you may have a short temper, be easily overwhelmed and frustrated, experience increased physical sensitivity, become hypervigilant, or struggle with intrusive thoughts. This is what I was contending with when I had flashbacks in the gym. When Kenny reminded me of "conditions first," I would center my focus on my body and my resources in an attempt to position myself in my window of tolerance before I lifted something heavy.

Hypoarousal is the opposite of hyperarousal. In this state, you may experience emotional and/or physical numbness, have reduced physical movement, feel frozen, lose time, and feel spaced out. When you are lying in bed or on your couch doomscrolling and you lose track of time and sort of forget to eat, shower, or go to sleep, you may have moved into a hypo-aroused state. Hypoarousal often feels like you simply cannot get up and do a darn thing.

Anyone can become overwhelmed, but the amount of stress it takes to push you there depends on your window of tolerance. Doing healing work and changing your physiology through things like strength training (which includes training your nervous system) is possible at the edges of the window of tolerance. In that transition zone, you're looking for a balance between experiencing discomfort and being able to stay present with the feelings, sensations, memories, and connections you trigger while doing this work. That's how you make your window a little wider and become better able to handle stressors.

Imagine if you showed up to physical therapy session for help with a back injury and the first thing you were instructed to do was pick something heavy up off the floor. If you were lucky, you might be able to lift it once without getting hurt. That's because you'd be attempting to heal from outside your window of tolerance, which is virtually impossible in physical and emotional therapy. A more mindful approach to your back injury might involve movement with gentle resistance, maybe from soft elastic resistance bands. That kind of work is hard, but not too hard—well inside the window. By not overwhelming your nervous system, all systems in the body can continue to perform their regular job even while engaged in the work of healing your back.

This principle remains true in talk therapy as well. A gentle approach to processing your trauma means slowing down, working with one piece of the story at a time, and then pausing to integrate that tolerable amount of important work. If you find yourself repeating a painful story over and over again, whether in counseling or to friends and loved ones, and being flooded with the same old feelings as if you were stuck in that moment, you are likely overwhelmed. This means that when your brain tells the story, the meaning-making, fear-quieting part of your brain is offline. The prefrontal cortex cannot do its job by helping you process that old and upsetting event so that you can integrate it into your past experiences, as opposed to reliving it as if it's happening in the present.

EXPLORING YOUR WINDOW OF TOLERANCE

Talking of being overwhelmed and having the limbic system call the shots brings up another question: How can you get your prefrontal cortex back online? As luck would have it, Dan Siegel also came up with a clever and portable model of the three-part, or "triune" brain, and "flipping the lid," which is what happens in your brain when you are overwhelmed; this is a useful shorthand to discuss moving in and out of our window of tolerance.

Look at your hand with your palm facing you, then make a fist with your thumb tucked in and fingers curled over your thumb. Now imagine your wrist is the brainstem, your tucked-in thumb is the limbic system, and your curled fingers are your prefrontal cortex. You have recreated a model of the triune brain. To illustrate what it's like when the prefrontal cortex is offline, lift up the four fingers curled over your thumb—this is your limbic system now at the helm, even if there is no actual threat to safety. This "lid flip" happens whenever you move beyond your window of tolerance and your prefrontal cortex goes offline.

The good news is that you can flip your lid back on with relative ease, reawaken the prefrontal cortex, and come back into your window of tolerance by using movement. My go-to technique is quite simple. I ask my clients to pass a ball back and forth between their hands across their midline, which requires you to redirect your focus to the movement at hand (literally), bringing both the right and left sides of your neocortex online and in touch with each other. In the Take Action below, I will walk you through the specifics of this regulating exercise.

Another technique involves playing with balance. "Play" is a key word here—you don't want to add pressure to an already over-whelmed system. Play is opt-in, casual, and fun, but still constructive. It integrates the analytic and creative parts of our brain with different bodily systems, allowing us to feel more at ease. One of my favorite pieces of gym equipment that I own is a portable balance beam. This nine-foot-long piece of purple foam rolls up so I can carry it in a big green tote bag. It's basically a giant toy, which my clients associate with play. At only two inches high, many people find walking on it to be challenging but doable—a non-threatening exercise. Whether you move across it by going forwards or backwards, you need to pause and pay attention before proceeding, and in that pause your prefrontal cortex "flips" back on.

Every person's skill level (with the beam or any other exercise) is different, and what constitutes playing with balance will look different to you than to the next person. For most people, a narrow, staggered stance is challenging on any surface, which is why I like the balance beam. But you could try more formal approaches, like variations of Tree Pose in yoga, in which you stand on one leg, or else improvise with what you have lying around. Maybe try balancing a ball or book on your hand or head. You may even find that there is space in there to get a little silly.

Simply calling to mind someone or something that supports you can also help you come back into your window of tolerance. After doing some movement, think of one of the resources you listed in your self-intake in the Take Action from the Introduction. Your body and mind may find some ease when you think about them.

I still find it very taxing on my nervous system when I train in weightlifting now, and it can push me toward the edge of my window of tolerance. But I don't worry that much about flipping my lid and going too far. First of all, I know how to come back from it; and second, even if I am not training with Coach Kenny, I can still call everything he taught me to mind by reminding myself, "conditions first."

TAKE ACTION
Passing the Ball Back and Forth

People often ask me what to do if you find yourself becoming so overwhelmed that you have a panic attack or flashback, while working out or at any other time of day. In times like those, I think it's best to have a simple tool at the ready that you can rely on just about anywhere. This is my go-to. While the name implies you need a ball on hand, any non-breakable object about the same size as a tennis ball will do.

This exercise can be used when you have "flipped your lid", but also to bring yourself more into your window of tolerance when you are enduring stress of any kind. I often use this technique between challenging sets in the gym.

WHAT YOU WILL NEED:
A tennis or lacrosse ball, or some other non-fragile object of comparable size

DURATION:
1 to 2 minutes

1. I invite you to stand and feel your feet on the ground, or sit and feel your seat on the chair, bench, or floor. Hold the ball in your hands. Check in with yourself and notice any thoughts, feelings, or sensations you might be experiencing. Don't change anything, just notice it.
2. Next, pass the ball from hand to hand across the middle of your body. You can think of it as switching hands or even a small toss. You want it to be just challenging enough to require some focus but not so challenging that there is a risk of dropping the ball with each toss. You don't want to add any additional frustration to the mix.
3. After a minute or two, pause. Check in again and notice any changes in your system. Has your breathing, posture, or any tension in your body shifted? What about how you feel emotionally? Are you more grounded? What is the speed of your thoughts?

Notice what shifts you were able to create with this small, simple movement.

4. Note that if you are using this technique in response to feeling overwhelmed, you can skip the initial check-in, which may in fact be more activating. Instead, start right away with passing the ball back and forth, and then after a minute or two check in and notice any shifts.

CHAPTER TWO

Shifting Your Relationship with Your Body

"**L**INE UP! CLASS IS OVER," my gym teacher hollered after blowing his whistle. It was a wrap on fifth grade gym class for the day. We were in a circle around our teacher, whom I cannot picture in any detail. All I remember was that, like most of my gym teachers, he was a white guy with a whistle who paid little attention to me. The gym at John F. Kennedy Middle School in Great Neck, Long Island, was big, its shiny wooden floors covered in stripes demarking sports-related things that I never quite understood. I traced the lines with my eyes, thinking about who knows what. I did not like looking up at my classmates.

Eric, from the other side of the circle of students, yelled, "C'mon, Laura. Sing!"

I was jolted out of my thoughts. I looked up and across the circle at Eric. What was he talking about? *I don't sing.* He was tall and skinny, with long limbs and thick, curly blonde hair that gave him added height. His face frequently bore an impish sort of expression that made his meanness read as "fun!" Standing there now with that face, he was clearly relishing whatever he was going to say next.

"It's not over 'til the fat lady sings!" he explained, erupting in laughter. I don't remember what my other classmates did, or if the teacher said anything. I do remember that I was flooded with shame, heat creeping up my neck to my ears and a wave of nausea passing through my guts. I wished I would just disappear. My eyes, now wet, went back to tracing the lines on the floor, but none led to the door I wanted to run through.

While I assume my corporeal form did not actually vanish at any point, I was gone in another sense. I dissociated. It was around this age that I really began to try to vanish, especially in the gym or at recess. No one in my memories from fifth and sixth grade has a clear face, and the little I remember is either from a bird's eye view or just a feeling. I remember Eric's face though, because he began picking on me in third grade, before my memories started to fade.

Bullies like Eric weren't the only people who made me feel that my existence was of less value than that of a thin person. I heard it in the way family members would talk about their own fatness or thinness. I saw it on television and read it in the fashion magazines I began to gobble up and swallow down during puberty, along with reduced-fat cookies and Slim Fast shakes. American culture, as reflected in what we consume and say to one another, reveals a pervasive problem of weight stigma and fatphobia.

Weight stigma, which entails negative attitudes toward fat people, is insidious, systemic, internalized by all of us, and directly leads to fatphobia. As of 2019, weight loss was a steadily growing $78 billion industry in the U.S.,[1] and the number of people going on specific diets that require restrictive eating is growing annually, despite the fact that multiple studies have shown that diets rarely work in the long term. Like other social stigmas, weight stigma and fatphobia are deeply harmful. People living in larger bodies are often regarded as lazy or less conscientious, and are written off as hopeless, unemployable, or likely to fail. Who wants to try something new—like walking into the gym or engaging in other healthy behaviors—if the message being sent to them is that they are likely to fail?

Weight stigma even impacts our healthcare system. One paper, reviewing the impact of weight bias on outcomes for obese patients, noted that physicians' biases led to less patient-centered care for obese clients, less time spent treating obese clients, and an over-attribution of symptoms and problems to obesity, rather than testing or treating actual underlying health problems.[2]

Given that it is culturally acceptable to make a person in a bigger body feel less likely to succeed, or less valuable, or loveable than their thinner counterparts, it's understandable that I spent a lot of energy worrying about what other people thought of my body, and how they were going to respond to it. I wasn't alone. Forty to sixty percent of girls aged six to twelve are concerned about their weight, or becoming "too fat."[3] Eric was the first of many people who would relentlessly bully me, going after my body. This made going to the gym emotionally loaded even as a teenager and young adult. To me, the gym was where the Erics of the world had free rein to mock, tease, and publicly shame. In turn, I associated the place with feeling less deserving of love and kindness than others. So I rarely went, and if I could have gotten away with never stepping foot in any sort of gym I would have. But my body had other plans for me.

I invite you to pause and check in. Consider giving yourself a hug.

When I was twenty years old, my back went out for the first time. I was working in the Mount Holyoke College archives for the second summer in a row—an air conditioned, on-campus gig working with primary source material—an American history nerd's dream summer job. I loved it. Was I lifting heavy boxes of famous women's writings when I hurt myself? Unfortunately, no. It was nothing remotely cool. My back went out as I got up from my desk chair after doing some totally unglamorous data entry. As I moved to stand from the chair, I felt my whole lower back seize, sending a sharp electric pain down my left leg and causing every other muscle in my body to tense up. I stood there, hunched, startled, and rigid. I immediately learned that if you cannot move your back, you cannot move your body. I was embarrassed and afraid. My body was so bad, I thought, that I threw my back out doing something as magnificently boring as getting up from a chair.

My mother took me back home to New York to see an orthopedic surgeon, who prescribed me physical therapy followed by exercise to heal the injury and get stronger. After spending a decade of my time and so much energy avoiding the gym, sports, and even being present in my body, I was very out of shape, weak and easily winded. As the doctor never said anything about losing weight, he earned my trust by showing faith in my ability to get stronger just as I was. So, I begrudgingly followed his recommendations.

I went to physical therapy the rest of the summer. Over the next several years, I would manage flare-ups by running on the elliptical in the gym while seething with self-loathing, worrying about people judging me for having the nerve to show up there so out of shape (which rarely helped my pain). I would think, "I'm too fat to go to the gym." None of these stopgap measures made me strong enough to get rid of my back pain altogether.

It would be another seven years before I met Ed Williams, the trainer who taught me that exercise could heal my back. But Ed did more than help me get me out of my back pain. Combining his technical skills as a trainer and coach with his commitment to being non-judgmental, his protective nature, his massive stature, and his even bigger heart, he would create the space and give me the tools to learn firsthand that I could do amazing things with my body, and undo a lot of the pain inflicted on me by diet culture.

This gym was an independent trainer gym (in other words, each person working out was there with a trainer), and I didn't feel it was safe for people existing in anything other than able and lean bodies. Some of the trainers were complete Erics and most were prone to at least some Eric-esque behavior. I would overhear them speaking disparagingly about folks on the floor, or even other trainers. Women were torn down for what they wore: "Who does she think she is, wearing that?

Ugh. Training in just a sports bra is a privilege, not a right." They would declare each other to be "fat," their voices dripping with vitriol as they dropped the f-bomb. Keeping in mind, they were leaner than anyone I had met before.

Overhearing these conversations made me nervous that they were taking jabs at me when I was out of earshot on the gym floor, and old feelings of wanting to vanish would stir. The whole atmosphere was damaging to my mental health and wellness and threatened to push me out of the gym again, a place where, according to my doctor, I should have been improving my health.

But knowing that I would see and work with Ed, who never equated how I looked with my value, was enough for me to be brave, show up, and get to work. Lifting would take me out of my head and my worries about other people's perceptions of me, and put me back into my body. Our sessions were generally grounding and became a source of pride. If I couldn't shake something I'd heard elsewhere in the gym, I would tell Ed. He would shake his head in disappointment at his colleagues. I know there were times when he gave other trainers a talking to. I hated those moments of feeling less than while I was there, but they were outweighed by the moments of feeling greater than I had previously thought myself capable of.

Big Ed made a big space for me to unpack a lot of the limiting internalized beliefs I had absorbed over the years. His point of view was that exercise is good for so much more than the things we can see. Like the orthopedist, Ed never made me feel that my weight made me less likely to take good care of my back. Nor did he carry a bias against people based on weight. My weight didn't make him think I was less capable of training, nor less worthy of his time and space in the gym. Ed is a true health and wellness practitioner. He is not blinded by weight stigma and understands that exercise is good for all sorts of systems you don't see, like your endocrine, cardiovascular, and nervous systems. Exercise boosts your mood, releasing neurotransmitters like dopamine and endocannabinoids, which produce that exercise high. It's empowering to set performance goals and reach them. It can help you manage chronic pain. And it can be fun! Yup. Gym class was not fun for me, but the gym can be fun.

In May 2020, as I was writing this chapter, I was shocked to come across an article penned by actor Matt McGorry breaking down the toxicity of diet culture. You may know McGorry from shows like *Orange Is the New Black* and *How to Get Away with Murder*. I knew him as a standoffish and chiseled trainer from the Chelsea gym. He wasn't an Eric, but he wasn't welcoming either. We shared space at the gym while he was filming, but after I'd seen the first two seasons of *Orange Is the New Black* and he'd stopped coming, he faded from my thoughts. So you can imagine my surprise when I came across an Instagram video of a sweet-looking, chubby, bearded McGorry talking with worried excitement about his vulnerable new article. This was not the reserved, chiseled trainer-cum-actor I knew from my gym. This was a wonderfully messy and vibrant human baring a vulnerable piece of himself. I liked what I saw, but was very confused. When had McGorry become an activist?

In the article, he wrote about being teased for being chubby as a kid and celebrated for being lean as an adult—one who would starve himself and beat his body into submission. He captured some moments from the gym when I knew him, but from a cisgender, white, lean, male trainer's perspective. The article validated my own experience in dealing with the Erics since childhood. Unlike me, McGorry had dealt with them in Hollywood, too.

But what really excited me was reading how this former trainer, whose potential judgment I'd feared, agreed with me on needing to get fatphobia out of gyms so they can be places of joyful movement, health, and wellness. He astutely writes,

> *"[F]itness, as we often use the term, tells us virtually nothing about how fit we are to complete certain tasks. When we say someone is "fit," it's almost never because we saw them demonstrate said fitness, but because they have a certain body type that leads us to assume what they can or can't do. These industries aren't selling fitness, but*

the promise of a socially acceptable body. Rather than the "fitness industry," we should call it the "thinness/leanness industry." An accurate name for the goals we're pursuing would at least force us to be honest about what we value: thinness and leanness, not health and wellness. If the reverse were true, we would focus on the fact that we undermine people who are trying to move their bodies and eat intuitively for their well-being when we make intentional weight loss a goal."[4]

When I became a trainer, I brought Ed's philosophy with me: the gym can be a place to find joy and empowerment. In recent years, I've been seeing more diverse and body-positive fitness professionals who, like me, got sick of the exclusionary and toxic fitness culture, and decided to break down the gates of the fitness industry, bang our pots and pans, and make change from within. They often identify as "body positive" or "health-at-every-size aligned." They make space for transgender people, non-binary people, and cisgender people alike; for people with fat bodies and people with skinny bodies; for people of color and white people; and for people who are able-bodied or living with a disability. Having all those people together in the gym is so exciting. These trainers recognize how harmful it is to sell fitness using weight stigma and fatphobia.

When I have spoken up in the past to mainstream fitness club owners about how diet culture in the industry, and in their spaces, is problematic, I am often met with the argument, "but it sells." "What does it sell, and at what cost?" I respond. My UK-based colleague and a Health At Every Size (HAES)-aligned trainer, Karen Preene, can always be counted on to give an honest answer that cuts straight to the point when asked for her perspective on fitness culture. So, I asked her if she thought selling gym memberships using fatphobic techniques was harmful. She said it was, "because it teaches people to associate exercise and movement with weight loss." She continued, "it conditions people to believe that the only valuable reason to exercise is to achieve weight loss. This belief often prevents people from establishing a long-term and intuitive relationship with exercise and movement. The relationship becomes reactive rather than supportive. People will often disengage if they don't achieve the desired result [weight loss], or they may develop a disordered relationship with exercise, attempting to maintain any weight loss achieved. The overall health aspects of exercise and movement are overlooked within diet culture."

It's wonderful that more and more fitness professionals and studios are carving out space for all bodies to exercise and move. But as individuals, we still have to do the heavy lifting of unpacking the harmful messages we all carry for us to begin engaging in embodied movement. Like Karen said, in a fatphobic world, people are likely to give up on exercise when they don't reach weight loss goals. But embodied movement, which is a more holistic path, is all about really experiencing our bodies, no matter how marginalized they may be.

It is hard to experience your body when you hate being in it. My fifth-grade self could have told you as much. We need to take steps to get through the hurtful self-talk that we have let take over our voices— our own true voices. We didn't know that bullying voice when we were little kids just being in our bodies, thinking we belonged wherever we were. That is, until someone told us, "you are not welcome here," (whether subtly or harshly, directly or indirectly).

It wasn't until I met another kid—this time, my own daughter— that I was able to silence the inner Eric who tore me down for my appearance. When I became pregnant with my daughter, I didn't want to see the world do to her what it had done to me: rob me of the joy of being in a human body regardless of how it presents. And I knew that would start with me treating myself with the sort of kindness that Ed had extended to me, and modeling that for my daughter.

TAKE ACTION
Reflect on the Habit of
Negative Self-Talk

Negative self-talk about your body undermines your efforts to heal. Healing requires some self-compassion, and your internal Eric makes it damn near impossible to be kind and gentle with yourself. This habit of kindness is actually a daily practice in *not* doing something—in this case, not saying mean things to yourself. It sounds odd at first, but this is how I began to undo the damage from bullies and make space for self-acceptance and love.

WHAT YOU WILL NEED:
A mirror, preferably one that allows you to see your whole body at once
A journal or a piece of paper
A writing instrument

DURATION:
5 minutes a day for at least 21 days

1. After you get dressed in the morning or near the start of your day, perhaps after some self-care, look at yourself in the mirror for about thirty seconds, and notice your thoughts about what you see.
2. If you have a positive thought, say it aloud to yourself and take a moment to notice any feelings that come up.
3. If you have a negative thought then acknowledge that you had a negative thought, but don't repeat it.
4. Take up to four minutes to record your experience and any meaning or observations you make of it.
5. If you are in therapy, it may be helpful to process the experience of doing this exercise with your therapist.

CHAPTER THREE

Examining Your Workout Baggage

I HAVE A COMPLICATED RELATIONSHIP WITH BAGS. I've carried one for as long as I can remember. As a child, I would pack my "toy bag" to go most places. It generally contained art supplies and my favorite stuffed dog, Brandon, who I still have tucked away in my tiny art room today. As an adult, I am often found toting around a gym bag or giant purse, which gives me the same guarantee of containing all that I could possibly need.

I don't really want to carry around all that stuff. I love the times when I can leave the house without my phone, keys, or wallet, but those are few and far between. So, since I have to carry stuff, I want my bag to look good and serve me well while I do it.

We all have our own personalities and our own needs. Although I am not a scientist (just a humble bag-and-practical-stuff enthusiast), I have a very "scientific" theory about this, and it has to do with bags: the ones we choose reflect our personality, and the things we carry in them reflect our needs. A tote bag showing support for a local PBS station sends a different signal than a tote bag that says "Balenciaga". That's not to say that they couldn't both belong to the same person, but each says something different.

My gym bags and their contents have always reflected my outlook on training. I used to feel ashamed of my body and just wanted to disappear from the gym, and for a while I all but did. My bags were nondescript and the clothes inside a sort of bland, uniform afterthought that helped me feel invisible. Later on, when I saw working out as a punishment for my "bad body," my bags were heavy and the clothes inside were designed to suck me in and strap down every jiggle when I jumped. But over time, my outlook has shifted far enough to see strength training as something I get to do, not have to do. My bags now are beautiful and full of brightly colored equipment that helps me lift heavy things.

We call our emotional trauma "baggage" for a reason. (Mine, I joke, is a matching set in a bold floral print, which includes a hat box, train case, and steamer trunk.) Each of us has our own emotional burden that we take with us from place to place. All our "stuff" is packed up in this body of ours, ready to go at a moment's notice—whether we feel like carrying it or not. Over time, I've been able to streamline my emotional baggage, making it lighter. And even though I still don't like schlepping it, I am strong enough to carry it with me most days.

I don't remember all of my past bags, nor do I remember everything I once carried in my emotional baggage, but I do remember the brown suede backpack I used in 1992. I was fourteen and had just enrolled at Fieldston, an upscale liberal private school in Riverdale, a Bronx neighborhood just north of Manhattan whose large single-family homes and abundant trees gave it a suburban feel. I was excited to be going there; the beautiful campus, with its nineteenth-century stone buildings dotting picturesque hills, made a nice change from the mid-century linoleum boxes I had attended up until then in New York's suburbs. It also had a strong arts program and the student body embraced the prevailing '90s grunge look, which really suited me. *Finally*, I thought to myself as I surveyed my new classmates, *a school where I can just dress the way I want to.*

I wore oversized flannel shirts, black crushed velvet maxi dresses, and the tallest Doc Martens I had time to lace up in the morning. You know that girl, or at least remember some version of her from high school—you probably read that description and thought "goth," or some other rebellious aesthetic.

But what you wouldn't have known then, is that "that girl" (me) led a dual life. Throughout middle school, I spent weekdays and every other weekend living with my father and stepfamily in Westchester, a suburb just north of New York City. When I was there, I dressed like a label-conscious mallrat, all in the hope of fitting in. But that never happened. Quite the opposite, in fact.

Something about me caught the attention of the mean girls, popular kids, "queen bees" or whatever you want to call them, and I spent eighth grade navigating an onslaught of bullying that left me with a complex I'm still unpacking today. By the end of eighth grade, I had a Pavlovian response to the telephone ringing, fearing yet another prank call intended to humiliate me. I dealt with threats of physical violence (girls moving to shove me down stairs and boys reaching out as if to grope my breasts) and daily public ridicule. I spent most of the year being humiliated for sport.

When I got dressed in Westchester, I would feel my anxiety increase. "Maybe today they won't notice me. Maybe today I'll dress right and they won't pick on my body," I would think. Dressing for Westchester stressed me out, which meant the mere act of getting dressed pushed me closer to the edge of my window of tolerance, decreasing my tolerance for all the other stresses of teenage life.

I invite you to pause, check in, and move part of your body even just a little bit.

There were breaks though. I spent every other weekend in New York City with my mother. When I was there, I wore her combat boots, my own oversized t-shirts and dark dyed jeans. New York City-me was a more comfortable me. My clothes were comfortable and since there was no school involved, I never had to be in a room full of my peers laughing at me; it was just me, my mom and her partner. I enjoyed getting dressed when I woke up in my mom's house. I never dressed in my city clothes when I was in Westchester because I thought too many people would notice, and I was desperately trying to remain unseen. Even then, a part of me knew that when we dress for ourselves, it feels better than when we dress for others.

By high school, New York City-me was a full-time gig. After my father divorced my stepmother, we left the suburbs and moved to midtown Manhattan, and I started at Fieldston. My mother described my style going into high school as "different—just like everybody else." I think this is what we want as adolescents, and even as adults. We want to be ourselves, and we want to be accepted, which often means that when we are being ourselves we are also looking a lot like our peers.

I liked how at Fieldston I was simultaneously able to be me and to blend in, comfortable in whatever I had on. Blending in was needed in Westchester, as it seemed like a safe way to get through school. I had left behind a life of conformity where I did not fit in at home or school, and traded it in for a more lowkey conformity that worked for me.

There was one exception to this: Fieldston had a *gym uniform.* This uniform made my whole body tighten up so hard twenty-five years ago that I still grimace when I think about it now. On the first day of school, I arrived in the gym, where a school store had been set up so we could buy textbooks, Fieldston swag, and much to my dismay, a gym uniform. I surveyed the room. Lines of kids who I did not yet know were chatting together. I looked down, embarrassed I didn't have anyone to chat with, and the all too familiar stripes on the gymnasium floor pulled my eyes until I had the courage to look up once more.

I moved toward the tables full of things I would need to carry for the year. I picked up my books. They were heavy, but something about new books has always sparked a joyful sense of promise inside me. So, bolstered by this excitement, I turned toward the gym uniform table. I moved slowly, as if approaching a wounded wild animal that might attack.

Laying before me was a pile of the shortest short-shorts I'd ever seen. To add insult to injury, they were Crayola orange with white piping. Orange makes me look, well, very orange. To the left of them were more piles of orange—t-shirts with white lettering and a big white square where we were supposed to write our names, and orange sweatpants with "Fieldston" written on the thigh in small lettering, also with a space to write your name. At the very end, there were some navy tees with orange letters. I had never been so happy to see navy blue.

I looked at those shorts, the shortest of shorts, and my skin flushed and burned. My stomach dropped. Just the thought of revealing that much of my legs started a geyser of shame that bubbled in my guts and threatened to spill hot tears from my eyes. I didn't know it, but I was teetering at the edge of my window of tolerance as an avalanche of thoughts showered over me.

You cannot wear those. You are too fat. No one will like you. They will be mean to you. You cannot wear those shorts. They won't even fit. You are too fat to be a person. You are too fat for friends. No one is going to like you here.

My brain gathered speed as it hurled insults. I was really good at being very mean to myself.

How could this new school, which had promised to be a safe haven from bullies, do this to me already? At fourteen, I had no idea that this was the voice of trauma: the trauma of being bullied in gym class by Eric and later others, in many other classes, and on the school bus, too. I felt personally threatened, but in reality, this attack hadn't happened and the uniforms were just dated leftovers from the '80s that none of the students liked. I didn't realize yet that I had brought those bullies with me in my emotional baggage, that their taunts and my own cruel thoughts were being carried in my body everywhere I went.

*I invite you to pause, check in,
and notice your surroundings.*

Thinking quickly on my feet, I bought two pairs of sweatpants and two navy shirts and got out of the gym as quickly as I could. I didn't buy the shorts, even though I wanted some so I didn't sweat too much in class. Instead, I cut one pair of sweatpants into shorts of a length I was comfortable with. (Creativity has always been a great personal resource of mine.) I left the squares for my name blank. Naming myself would call too much attention to my existence.

When I showed up to gym class, unnamed and in my cut-offs, no one said a thing. Either the alterations were permissible, or I'd succeeded in becoming one with the bleachers, not even the teachers able to see me as I vanished. For someone who thought they were too big, I was very good at becoming invisible.

Regardless of my creative problem-solving and the relief that people didn't make fun of me in gym class, my altered gym uniform became a totem of my body shame, and I resented having to be responsible for it. On top of having to claim and wear this uniform, I also had to remember to bring it home regularly to wash it and bring it back to school. This was like salt in the wound. Every time I looked at those clothes, sweaty or clean, they reminded me of how much I hated my body. And they were almost always with me in my school bag, a brown suede Jansport backpack that I otherwise loved.

CLAIMING—AND REPLACING—YOUR BAGGAGE

For my friends who knew me in high school, seeing images of me over twenty years later on my personal training website in designer athleisure, hauling my gym bag with all my gear for strength sports on the subway, must have been a hoot. Having to carry anything gym-related, no matter how deep I shoved it into my book bag, used to send me down a spiral of shame. Nowadays, I can tell you my favorite manufacturer of workout tights, sports bras, gym bags, sneakers, and all manner of gear, and I am proud to be seen in gym clothes. I was so proud of these photos that were a testament to my feeling awesome about my body, particularly in the gym.

As someone who has always loved clothes and shoes and who now loves to work out and train, I get pretty excited about activities that require specialized athletic wear. Olympic weightlifting is one of those sports with "special shoes." They have a raised heel to help you get into a good position at the bottom of a lift, provide you with a solid base, and support your feet to help you as you lift. They are sometimes referred to as lifters, or weightlifting shoes. These shoes were the first piece of gym equipment I ever bought that made me feel like it might somehow be okay if someone actually noticed me in the gym. Unlike my ugly and unflattering Fieldston gym uniform, these shoes, I decided, made me look like a badass. In my internal narrative, people who wear weightlifting shoes are strong and brave enough to catch at least thirty-three pounds of steel over their head, again and again.

Ultimately, it was Olympic weightlifting that would finally allow me to drop my high school baggage—wanting only to shrink my body, disappear, and have no one know my name in the gym—and pick up a new, amazing bag to celebrate that, for the first time since puberty, I felt good in my body when I practiced something physical.

I wasn't great at weightlifting, but I felt strong and I was learning how to move in a new way. The sport demands you know where your body is in space as you move it around a barbell that you have powerfully driven into the air, so I was cultivating greater physical awareness. It also demanded that I pay attention to how it felt as I moved through the lift. Without knowing it, I had begun to lay the groundwork of an embodied movement practice. And as I did all of that, in the background, I was unpacking the baggage of being bullied in middle school.

I had been squatting and deadlifting to build my strength when I ordered my shoes. I did some research and learned that Pendlay Do-Wins are known to fit a wider foot like mine. (Yes, at the time I even had body shame about my slightly wide feet.) When my package came, I immediately opened the box and tried them on. They were white, purple, and black with black soles. I showed them off to my husband and daughter the way someone might show off a pair of red-soled Louboutins. They fit and I placed them in my gym bag—a bag that must have been practical yet very unexciting, because I cannot for the life of me remember what it looked like. This was a case of the contents mattering more than the bag.

I showed up at the gym with my special shoes and Big Ed took it as a signal that I was mentally prepared to give Olympic weightlifting a shot. So, that was the day I began to learn how to do a snatch, the lift in which you move the bar from the ground into the air, catching it in a squat overhead.

I loved those shoes. They became imbued with so much meaning. So much so that by putting them in my gym bag, I had transformed it into a symbol of just how awesome I was. I was a weightlifter.

A NEW WAY TO PACK

When it comes to doing hard work and lifting heavy things, some of you may have to lift less, and some of you, like me, will have to lift more. What you keep with you to tend to your needs changes with your activities, priorities, and self-perception. But we all have needs. That's why we carry gym bags or keep our exercise supplies tucked away together at home, perhaps in a basket in a corner of our living room or on a shelf in our garage.

My needs changed over time. At first, I packed to be unnoticed. Although it didn't feel good, that's what I needed to do to show up and, in time, start lifting heavy things. Being able to disappear was a resource. Remember, that was how I made it through fifth grade, middle school, and high school PE, not to mention college PE, too. When I found a resource to replace invisibility—in my case, Ed—I was able to shed that behavior. But at first, training was also just a habit, and my bag was just a thing I carried. Then I found a sport I loved, and my bag became stuffed with heavy gear, but also with the joy I found in training. That resource—pride and strength in my body—made me love my gym bag and propelled me to keep going to the gym.

At some points as these needs shifted, they felt like a lot to carry. But now I know that's not a reflection that I myself was ever "too much." I want to tell you, my friend, that you are never too much. Maybe that's what your family or friends told you, or what society told you through advertising, media, and social media. But you are not too much.

Regardless of how much stuff you carry, literal or metaphorical, you are certainly not being too much by giving yourself the resources you need to take care of yourself. Resources are a fundamental condition to do the work of lifting heavy things. They make you feel safe and prepared to approach the edges of what you can tolerate, knowing that you have the supports to do so.

TAKE ACTION
Unpacking and Repacking

My workouts have changed over the years and what I need to support myself, in a practical sense, has changed along with them. Whatever you carried in your real or metaphorical gym bag in the past may not be what you need today. Giving yourself practical equipment that suits your needs while you work out and thereby supporting yourself and your movement practice is an act of self-care.

During the intake, you took stock of the conditions you need to practice movement, which includes gear.

Along with that list, there are a handful of other items you might have overlooked or may want after you read this book. Below is a list of practical items I've pulled from experience to have on your person wherever you work out.

For any session, at home or away:

- A small massage ball
- If you have long hair, hair ties
- A journal and a writing instrument that you like, for recording reflections, your training plan, and anything else (you could add your goals and resource lists from page 15 here)
- A snack that provides you with protein and carbs
- A water bottle
- A favorite playlist and something to play it on
- A fitness plan or program
- Any other gear you may need to do your program or sport

If you work out at home, you might keep these items in a basket or bin wherever you exercise. If you work out in your kitchen or bathroom (yes, I know people who do this), perhaps there's some storage under the sink. If you work out in your living room or bedroom, you could tuck it away somewhere in a container that you like in your space.

For training away from home, like at a barbell club, YMCA, other fitness studio, or gym:

- Extra hair ties if you have long hair (and maybe want to help out another long-haired gym-goer)
- Toiletries and a change of clothes
- Headphones
- A little totem that reminds you of your favorite person or pet from outside the gym

If you are going to work out outside of your home, you'll need to pick a bag to use. This bag reflects both your purpose in using it and your personality. Start by considering whether you're the kind of person who doesn't mind having a gym bag, or if you see it as a burden. Do you have a car? Can you leave your stuff in the car? Or do you get around on foot and by public transportation? Can you rent a locker?

Once you know how much you are going to be carrying and where, it is time to consider the bag itself. Are you like the folks who need their bag to multitask, taking it to work and other engagements? Or can you keep your tote from your favorite bookshop, charity, public radio station or supermarket packed up and in your car? Do you want a backpack, a tote, or a duffel? Does it need to zip shut? How big should it be? Do you care whether you look cool? (I swear it is ok if your answer is yes. I care whether I look cool. Honor that about yourself and pick a bag that makes you feel cool, however you define this.)

Congratulations! You've taken a big step toward lifting heavy things, and toward healing, by understanding what you need to show up and feel supported as you do this hard, yet invaluable work. And remember: come back to your bag periodically to clean it out and check to make sure its contents still support your needs.

CHAPTER FOUR

Orienting to Your Space and Your Workout

I HAVE DONE A LOT OF HEALING WORK over the years, but that doesn't mean I am now without scars or that I don't still get triggered. During the spring of 2020, COVID-19 coverage had me spinning out multiple times a day. I felt like I did during the early days of living with PTSD. Panic would wash over me throughout the day, my stomach ached as if I had been punched in the gut, and my whole body shook. I squeezed my eyes shut, wishing I would disappear. Then I would shake my head, my shoulders, and my trunk. I would wiggle in my seat. And all that back and forth movement would flip my proverbial lid back on long enough for a thought to grab my attention. This was my Voice of Reason, which lives inside my prefrontal cortex—the me who had the tools I needed to tend to myself when I am triggered despite being safe.

"Look around, you are safe right here and now," the Voice assured me, time and time again. I would open my eyes and take in my surroundings. I might also listen for familiar sounds, breathe in the scent of the air around me, and place my hand on my belly, using touch to remind myself I am present. I was orienting.

Orienting is something you do instinctively under threat, but it can also be done intentionally when you need to come back to the present moment and demonstrate to yourself that you are safe. It's a tool you can use no matter where you are.

I used orienting techniques almost hourly that spring. Sometimes it was in a moment of distress, just to remind myself I was okay, and sometimes it looked more like familiarizing myself with a new space and identifying possible resources. (I had relocated to South Carolina without planning to.) Orienting to my new, temporary home was also my first step in making a home gym with no gym equipment so I could continue to strength train during what I knew would be a very trying time.

On March 20, New York Governor Andrew Cuomo put the state "on pause" in response to the virus's rapid spread. We were four days into our quarantine in South Carolina. I had already accepted that the pandemic was going to turn our world upside down, and I signed a lease on our rental so we could stay.

We spent the first two fear-filled weeks of quarantine in a beach-front condo, which created some dissonance. We had left New York thinking it would be a five-day vacation, but shortly after we arrived, we understood we would be staying longer. We were surrounded by vacation energy but haunted by pandemic turmoil. I would wake up and sit on our wooden balcony with my first coffee of the day, watching the sun rise over the Atlantic and shaking off the cobwebs of an anxious night's sleep as I admired the pelicans. They were big, with broad wingspans, and I was totally enthralled by their might and beauty as they flew fast, then dove with grace and power down toward the sea.

I showed up fully for these moments. I listened to the ocean, slowly syncing up with its steady rhythm; watched the birds and felt awe and joy despite my nerves, and eventually, I had a moment where I felt quiet on the inside. I was sad and even scared, but it was tolerable and I felt brave.

But over the course of each day, as if with the tide, my fear would rise with every reported case of COVID-19, and I worried about having enough toilet paper and food. By bedtime, I would be gripped with fear and lie rigid in my bed. I would listen for the sound of the waves crashing against the sand and, somehow, manage to fall to sleep. Despite being fitful, it was better than not sleeping at all.

I spent my days in the condo riding waves of anxiety, while simultaneously being charmed by the space. It looked like it was decorated by the Golden Girls, with its pastel and beige rooms filled with Formica and wicker; seashells filled glass lamp bases and sun-faded watercolor beach scenes adorned the walls. While this particular aesthetic is far from my own taste, my parents', or even my grandparents', it held a familiar nostalgia that woke up childhood me, who felt like she was on vacation. Sinking into the soft, overstuffed beige leather couch like it was the lap of a person with arms to contain me, I noticed that I could breathe in a way I hadn't been able to in New York. Each time thoughts of the virus took me away from my body, I would take in my surroundings and remind myself, *I am here right now, and right now I am okay.*

I invite you to pause, check in, and notice the
way you're being supported by the ground, seat,
or bed below you, and how this feels.

After a two-week quarantine, we moved to a slightly bigger house out of the resort and off the beach. I rented this place having only seen the online listing. I never met a manager or landlord. It had a keypad so we never even had to pick up the keys. It was clean, sweet, and welcoming—literally. When I first walked into the house, my eyes fell on a piece of wooden wall art, probably eighteen inches square: cedar planks, with a wooden silhouette of South Carolina and a heart in the middle painted cream, mounted above a teal-painted cut-out of the word "Home." Just past it, another wall hanging said, "Welcome to the beach." This place invited me in when I looked at it. It gave me hooks and a shelf: a place to hang my jacket, purse, and keys when I came home. I was relieved.

You could tell it had recently been redone by the absence of scuff marks on the walls and signs of use in the kitchen, beyond one scuffed-up pan. It had the calming neutrality-meets-brightness of an IKEA catalog and was full of decorative elements celebrating the local region. I fell in love with a vibrant painting of ten tall, skinny palm trees with blue water just beyond, beckoning me to an imaginary swim. That painting became my constant companion, visible over my shoulder in every Zoom meeting I took there.

When you encounter a new stimulus—which is anything unfamiliar that gets your attention, like a house or an animal or a person's face—you're naturally drawn to it. Think about when you hear a loud noise or something in your peripheral vision grabs your attention. What do you do? You turn toward and automatically assess the situation. When it's something sudden, you likely ask, "What was that?" Whether or not you actually verbalize it, you begin to look around to see if there is a threat present. You look to see how other people are reacting to it and take further cues from them. And then you act based on what you've discovered. If it was nothing, you return to your day. But if it's a threat, you mobilize. Surveying the scene is part of keeping yourself safe.

We all need to feel safe in our body and our environment in order to do healing work. Orienting, like resourcing, is one way you can achieve that. Although orienting out of surprise is an instinctual response, we can also intentionally orient to new spaces in order to promote a feeling of safety. We may look for resources or just get to know the lay of the land. This house was new to me, so I began checking it out room by room. Looking around, I felt calm when my eyes fell on pleasing things. Listening, I heard birds chirping and kids playing basketball across the street. I settled into my body and into the space.

Once we unpacked our bags, it was time to turn a 1,300-square-foot, three-bedroom house not just into a home, but a home office for two, a homeschool for one, and a home gym for three. I looked around, continuing to orient myself. I knew which resources we had, but I wanted to get a feel of which parts of the space might work best for each activity.

Once I'd determined where each of us would feel most comfortable and be able to meet our daily needs, I harnessed my creative superpowers yet again. Only this time, instead of making gym shorts that I could deem okay enough to wear, I was going to make an office with a desk for my daughter, two workspaces for my husband and I, and a gym that we could all use for the next two and a half months.

I moved furniture, tucking a dresser away into a closet and turning a side table into a desk by propping it up on cases of soda. (I'd purchased these on sale at the local Harris Teeter just to use them as risers!) My daughter now had a separate room with a door where she could attend school virtually.

I moved extra dining chairs around, repositioned the coffee table and a club chair in the living room, and either repurposed the decorative knick-knacks provided by our hosts to be used as training objects or tucked them away to make space for our own stuff. David and I set up workstations at the dining table and in the living room respectively. He had a firm chair and an ergonomic setup with good connectivity, and I had my preferred nest in a club chair with a side table-cum-desk.

Then it was time for me to make a gym. Knowing that I was set up to strength train would make me feel like I could really land in this home, and it would give each of us a space to get into our bodies and take care of ourselves indoors. We were taking this bright, neutral IKEA house and making it our home.

There was space in the living room for one person to work out at a time. With a yoga mat, two jugs of water, a broom, two more cases of soda, books, and a backpack, my husband and I were each equipped to continue our training routines. The water jugs worked like dumbbells or kettlebells on their own, or like barbell plates when slid onto each end of the broom. I used them for rows, swings, and one-arm snatches. Backpacks filled with books served as kettlebells, sandbags, and weight vests. I would wear it on my back for planks, and swing it around to the front for squats. I used cases of soda as a substitute for sandbags, as well as for single-handed overhead carries. Books on their own were light dumbbells used for shoulder stability work, or a step for me to use for calf raises. I placed a thin book under my heels to provide elevation while doing split squats.

I could not have made myself a gym if I hadn't taken the time to orient myself to the space. I had to get to know it a little. Intentional orienting is grounding. As you live your life, and especially if you are trying to live your life to the fullest, you are likely to encounter new spaces. But for some of us, unfamiliar new spaces may feel threatening. By intentionally orienting yourself, you can gather the information necessary for you to use the space as intended and to support your needs. This information, like the stuff in your gym bag, is another kind of resource, and it's part of putting the conditions in place to be able to do what you are there for.

I knew how to do this because I have helped many clients get set up in their own homes, from stay-at-home caregivers to people who didn't feel safe in the gym due to past trauma, or didn't have room in their budget for a gym membership. We would meet online via video, me looking around my home as they looked around theirs, and would figure out how to make this work for their life as it was, right then and there. Kitchen counters, IKEA step stools and stairs are all fair game for push-ups and step-ups. Bric-a-brac becomes weights. Kids become weights, too, as well as cheerleaders, DJs, and workout buddies.

ORIENTING—CREATING A SAFE SPACE FOR HEALING

No matter where you train, it can be helpful to not only orient yourself to the space, but also to your workout. You orient to a space by looking around and noticing where things are. If you're preparing to engage in movement at home, survey your space, whether it's a small studio or house with a garage and an extra room. Think about which part of the space best meets the conditions you feel you need to train. This might be zero clutter, privacy, or proximity to a Wi-Fi router. Get to know your home in the context of engaging in a movement practice. And when you choose somewhere to practice, be intentional with picking a place to store any equipment you need, too. Have a plan for setting up and putting away equipment if the space is multipurpose or shared with others.

When you walk into a gym, studio, or fitness center for the first time, take a moment to get to know where a few things are: equipment, bathrooms, and a place to leave your stuff. You might be the sort to ask to be shown around, or you might investigate yourself. Either works, but start to make a mental map of the place.

I also suggest that you orient yourself to the practice each day. By that, I mean considering what shape your practice is going to take. If you attend a class, chances are that it'll have a general framework. Before class, while everyone is setting up, you might ask the instructor or someone who has taken the class before about the general format. Fitness professionals generally come into the studio with a plan they can share with you. For those of you training on your own, a training journal can come in handy. Not only can you use it to track your workouts, but also to plan what you're going to do next. If you are designing your own routine, you can write (or draw) your program in your journal, or if you're following someone else's program, you could transcribe it in here with space for notes at the end. Knowing the plan is a way to orient to your practice on a daily basis.

Even though my work has involved writing strength training programs for other people, I don't actually write my own. When I'm following a personalized program from a trainer or a group program, I receive it in a spreadsheet or text document and then transcribe my program in my journal, using whichever format makes sense to me. I leave little blanks to add numbers of reps completed and weight used. Transcribing them by hand really grounds me in what I am going to be doing for the next hour or so.

When working one-on-one with a client, I provide them with the same information. For some in-person clients, I tell them verbally what to expect at the start of each session, while others prefer to have their own hard copy of the program so they can look at the program while we work. I help them read it if they're inclined to look; some clients prefer to see this information, and others prefer to hear it. In all cases, the senses are key in orienting to the practice. Some folks like to know how many reps they'll have to do, because not knowing how long they'll need to keep doing one thing can make training, which activates the nervous system, suddenly feel inescapable. Others don't want to know anything beforehand—my guess is that those people like having someone they trust around to take care of them and guide them through the stressors. Some people's preferences vary from day to day. And all these variations are perfectly normal to me. I'm pointing this out because people often ask, "Is it weird that I want to know?" or "Is it weird that I *don't* want to know?" To which I always say, "Nope. Not weird." Reviewing a workout plan is a form of orientation, and we all naturally orient ourselves to create the condition of safety. Who doesn't want to feel safe?

Sometimes we may know rationally that we are safe, but feel like we aren't. Using orienting techniques, you can assess the accuracy of these feelings in a given situation and be better equipped to leave the situation if you still don't feel safe. By creating an opportunity for your senses to tell your brain where you are, what's going on, and how safe it is, you are empowering yourself to be present and take up space.

I ground myself through orienting a lot, not just in the gym or when I travel. As a writer with a penchant for memoir, I often use it after I write. In order to bring my reader into my past more fully, I need to take myself out of the present and put myself back into the story I'm trying to tell. I often feel disoriented when I'm done with a writing session, and if I don't address it, I can become anxious. I close my computer and take some time to really look around my workspace. I take in my green laptop case, empty coffee cup, my hefty garnet the size of a tennis ball—an opaque, dark red with black veins. Then I look out the window to my right and notice the weather and time of day. I look into the kitchen to my left and notice if it is messy or clean. I check the time. I feel my breath.

I orient after I talk about painful memories in therapy, too, using techniques provided at the end of this chapter. I am sharing them with you so you can use them whenever you need to come back to the present from past memories, or recover from anxiety about the future.

Orienting yourself to a space through your senses creates a safe container in which you can more fully connect with new experiences, deal with the mundanities of everyday life, and do the work of lifting heavy things.

TAKE ACTION
Orienting to Your Space Through
Sight and Sound

You can intentionally orient through your senses anytime, anywhere. It takes a minute or less. While there are several grounding techniques that use orienting through the senses, I use two techniques for myself and clients: *Five Things* and *Sounds Near to Far*. Everyone is different, so for some of you, it will be easier to ground with sight and for others, with sound. Keep in mind that touch, taste, and smell can also be grounding, but are not always as readily accessible.

WHAT YOU WILL NEED:
Yourself

DURATION:
1 to 3 minutes

FIVE THINGS
This technique is particularly useful when you need to quickly come back to the here and now. I use this technique a lot in therapy and when I have become overwhelmed in public spaces.

- Look around for five blue things. Look not just in front of you, but to the left and right, behind you, above you, and below you. As you see them, name them.
- Repeat, but this time look for five yellow things.
- Repeat, but this time look for five red things.
- Repeat as needed with different colors, until you feel grounded in the present.

SOUNDS NEAR TO FAR

I bring my attention from the world inside me to the world around me using this ritual, at the end of many of my training sessions and other healing work.

- Sit or stand with a soft, downturned gaze, looking at nothing in particular, or with eyes closed. Listen to your own sounds: your breath, your stomach gurgles, the sound as you swallow.
- Now listen to sounds just outside of you. This could be the creaking of the building or someone else doing something nearby. Where are these sounds in relation to you?
- Next, listen to sounds even further away—perhaps from outside the building you're in. What do they tell you about what's going on outside? Perhaps it's raining or windy, or you're reminded that you're in the middle of a busy city.
- When you are ready, open your eyes or lift your gaze and take in the space around you.

PART II
ACTIVATION

Once you have the conditions in place to lift heavy things safely, you can begin to do the work more confidently. This will involve engaging in a bit of discomfort as well as nervous system activation.

CHAPTER FIVE
Fostering Your Mind-Body Connection

UNTIL I BEGAN TO PRACTICE Olympic weightlifting (as opposed to lifting weights for strength training), I spent most of my adult life mentally checked out of my body. It didn't feel safe there. Bullying, medical trauma, and uncomfortable feelings of anger, fear, and rejection that I experienced as a child and teenager stayed with me, making me want to disappear.

Dissociation was how I coped. I want to be clear here that dissociation should not be pathologized—it is a survival strategy. A problem arises when we cannot re-associate after the threat has passed. Emotionally, it means not being able to fully experience life: neither the pain, nor the joyful parts. Physically, it can lead to chronic pain and even injury. Dissociation can occur in the body as a whole, but in the gym, we fitness professionals often notice that clients are out of touch with one part of their body in particular. For example, it is much harder for me to intentionally flex the muscles on the left of my chest and upper back. Whenever I have rushed doing activation exercises intended to turn them on, I have experienced flashbacks in the form of intrusive thoughts and waves of fear of annihilation. Herein lies the problem: you need to find the sweet spot between reconnection, where you can protect your joints by

actively using all of your muscles, and overwhelm. One specific therapeutic modality, called Somatic Experiencing (or SE), taught me that
the best way to do this is slowly and thoughtfully, even if that kind of
movement is not usually associated with lifting heavy things.

In the fall of 2018, a young woman in her twenties (whom I'll call
Emma) came to me for help with feeling grounded as she engaged in
a lot of personal development work in therapy. She, like many of my
private clients, spent a lot of time in her head and she wanted to train
to feel more comfortable being present in her body. She specifically
wanted to cultivate a posture that allowed her to get through daily tasks
with greater ease and less pain. She had aches and pains throughout her
body, was not physically active, and wanted to add movement to her
wellness plan. Emma had a great sense of humor, was whip-smart, and
very personable with me and other folks at the gym. She always showed
up to train and rallied on the days she did not necessarily want to be
there. She liked that strength training was hard but could also be fun,
and that it left her feeling better and better over time.

At the beginning of our work together, I emphasized pulling exercises to address her postural goals and to help ease some of her discomfort. At first glance, she could mimic every pulling exercise quite
well, and if I hadn't really looked at her back while she moved, I may
have missed the signs that some of her back muscles were offline. On
taking a closer look, I noticed that her left upper back was slightly more
developed than her right. On her left, she was moving more efficiently,
pulling with her back and her arm, and showing awareness that a pull
not only involves your arm but parts of your trunk as well. But on the
right side, it appeared she was pulling with just her arm.

I'd seen this with other clients, where one muscle is underactive, so
another muscle becomes overactive to compensate. Our amazing and
resilient bodies do this dance, known as movement compensation, to
allow us to move about the world and get stuff done. Movement compensation can become habitual, establishing a mind-body connection
that says *this is how we have to execute this movement.* Ultimately, this can
create a cycle of over-compensation, leading to joint pain and injury.

Whenever I approach correcting my clients' muscle imbalances, we first go beyond the average warm-up, getting the heart pumping and body warm to encourage embodiment. I program activation exercises for sleepy muscles as part of my personal warm-up, and whenever I see the need for them in clients. Activation exercises are simple, in that they often isolate a single body part but get your whole nervous system going. When they are done correctly, you feel the targeted group of muscles working. They help establish a mind-body connection and change the way our nervous system mobilizes our muscles, bringing our offline muscles back online.

Once I noticed Emma's muscular compensation patterns, I introduced some activation exercises to see if they might help. I invited her to sit facing the seated rowing machine, legs stretched out before her, feet braced on the foot holds and arms extended, with her hands gripping the handles. From that position, I cued her to find both sides of her "lats," or *latissimus dorsi*, a large muscle that starts by the pelvis and spans up and along the back like an upside-down triangle, attached to the shoulders. The lats has many functions, including helping you pull while rowing.

"Squeeze your armpits like you're trying to squeeze orange juice with them." Her tank top left enough of her back bare that I could see her lats engage on both sides.

"Ok, now what?" she asked.

"Can you feel the muscles in your back? On both sides."

"I can feel it on my left," she answered.

"Is it okay if I touch your back?" I asked her in response.

"Yes." I tapped her right lat and then her left lat. I tapped her shoulders near her neck to make sure the wrong muscle wasn't engaged.

"Can you feel it now?"

"I can feel you tapping me." She could feel what was on her skin, but not what was going on below.

"Can you feel the muscle?" I asked. I could see it was working, or trying to, as it began to shake. She'd been squeezing for around fifteen seconds, so it was getting tired.

"No."

We kept this isometric hold as part of her warm-ups and, over time, we were able to slowly raise her awareness of her right upper back using activation drills, followed by embodied strength training. Slowly rebuilding a relationship with that part of her body was empowering, grounding, and allowed Emma to better handle daily tasks. She also experienced a reduction in her neck pain.

TRAUMA AND DISSOCIATION

So, why do muscles shut down in the first place? Trauma, physical or emotional, can be one reason. When you go through trauma, you may also have parts of your body shut down or have no sense of feeling in your body at all. On the other hand, you may find it hard to stay in your body, or a part of your body, through an entire range of motion, or even the complete contraction or extension of one particular muscle. I saw this time and again with clients and had also experienced it myself while training my upper back and chest.

According to Dr. Maureen Gallagher—a licensed psychologist and psychotherapist, as well as Somatic Experiencing Practitioner and one of my teachers from the Somatic Experiencing Trauma Institute—this phenomenon is called "undercoupling." She describes it as a "bottle-necking." In other words, it is the body saying, "too much, too fast, too soon. I can't process all this information and to deal with this too-muchness that's going on, I'm going to let go of some elements of my experience."

She's also talked about something most of us have encountered: people flattening their affect in speech. An example of this is some-body telling you a horrible, devastating story with a matter-of-fact tone, devoid of emotion—like saying that their mother died suddenly, but it's as if they were telling you about shopping for groceries. This is a form of dissociation. In this case, a dissociation of emotions from the events of the story. Not feeling the emotional effects of a traumatic incident has "survival value," as Dr. Gallagher noted. "Now you can walk through life and tell your story, and you're not bogged down by the feelings that go with that story, which were overwhelming to you."

As a personal trainer, I don't always know my clients' trauma history. The fact is, the 'why' is not so important for this work. I don't tell my story, partly to demonstrate this truth. What is important is that under-coupling, or the dissociation of a body part or the entire body, is occurring at all. I asked Dr. Gallagher in an interview for this book whether this dissociation happens in a particular body part because that part is linked to a traumatic event.

"Right. The mind is dissociating from that part of the body."

"Because people want to dissociate from that event?" I pushed.

"Or from pain itself," she explained. "Let's say your hand was harmed in a car accident. The body will produce natural analgesics (pain relief) to help you get through that event. But the numbing itself may continue longer than necessary, after the injury is healed. Also, it can be uncomfortable when you first return to sensation, and you might have a loop happening where when the natural analgesic decreases, the person feels pain, which then has the body producing more."

Compensatory movement habits can often be addressed in the gym with corrective exercise techniques, such as myofascial rolling and stretching of the muscles that were working too hard, activation of the muscles that were offline, and total body movements to get all the muscles working together. But if the cause of the shutdown is related to a trauma, you must go slowly and give your body time to adjust. If you don't, and don't listen to your body throughout this process, the system is easily overwhelmed. At best, no lasting change will occur, and at worst you can really push yourself outside your window of tolerance. Going slowly is the best way to ensure you create the changes you need in your system.

I invite you to pause, check in, and if it would feel
good to you, slowly roll your shoulders. Maybe even
allow your arms to join in the movement, too.

The topic of dissociation brings to mind another client, Sarah. During her intake, it became apparent that she used to spend more time pursuing physical interests but stopped at a certain point. When she came to me, she was very interested in pursuing different group fitness modalities. But she also had a lot of joint pain and felt she needed some individual help before engaging further in group fitness. Sarah was frustrated by instructors who would tell her to ignore the pain and discomfort she felt during class.

As we worked together, we were able to drastically reduce a lot of the joint pain in her lower body through hip stability work, but her upper back and shoulders presented a real challenge. When she focused her awareness there, she would not only feel the muscles but would become overwhelmed by muscle spasms. Going straight from dissociation to overwhelm is a common challenge faced by folks living with trauma. The good news is that by practicing muscular activation drills, you can slowly start to tap back into body parts you've been dissociated from. This will be a big support in your healing work and in strength training as well.

Dr. Gallagher described this scenario as moving "from nothing to too much," noting that this results from a combination of dissociation from the body part and an inability to titrate the experience of bringing it back online. In titration, Somatic Experiencing Practitioners (SEPs) help clients work through small and tolerable amounts of discomfort at a time. A technique known as *pendulation* is also used to combat this overwhelm. Pendulation involves moving your attention from places of discomfort in the body to neutral or good-feeling places. My time with Sarah came to a close before we really had the chance to work with titration, which is a slow and steady process requiring time and patience.

Before I started working with clients one-on-one, I worked at JDI Barbell as a Strength Groundwork coach, preparing clients to train for barbell sports. I noticed there was a handful of people who, when asked, could not tell me about bodily sensations they were feeling when they set up for a squat, bench, or deadlift.

This would sometimes lead to feelings of confusion or distress, but more often than not, these folks shrugged it off and kept going. As a coach, I continued to work with them on activation and bringing back feeling so they could learn to lift safely. But I drew the line there. Clients at JDI Barbell were coming to me to learn how to train with a barbell—not for trauma healing (though as I've realized, the therapeutic method was ingrained in all my training). Hopefully, as I did when I began to lift, they found some measure of healing anyway.

Perceiving the visceral feeling of a physical sensation inside the body is known as *interoception*. Accessing, or developing access to interoception is fundamental to allowing the possibility of healing trauma. As we continue to look at the other conditions needed to heal throughout this book, such as boundaries and agency, you will see how interoception is the cornerstone of each of these.

It has been my experience, both as a client and a witness, that in the gym, when some coaches or trainers are confronted with resistance—in the form of a lack of interoception, or even louder protests like tears and pain—they encourage their clients to just push through. Their intentions may be good but asking people to override their body's distress signals can cause harm. Pushing through resistance will almost always push folks out of their window of tolerance, even if done with their consent. Furthermore, in the case of folks who have had their boundaries breached and their sense of agency taken away due to trauma, pushing to override resistance can actually be retraumatizing. Resistance is information that should not go ignored, nor be overridden. It should be listened to and explored.

As much as there is information in resistance itself, I believe that there's even more in those places we don't want to explore—the parts of us we dissociate from. As a Somatic Experiencing Practitioner, I am curious about the parts of our bodies we cut ourselves off from, but I will only go there when the mind and body are ready. When I am working with a client and encounter a lack of interoception, I pause and assess how to help them slowly cultivate it. In that way, they can shift from resistant to curious. In SE, we arrive at this place gradually, using resourcing, titration, and pendulation. When we're ready to work with the dissociated parts, we want to work in *tolerable discomfort*—that is, discomfort that does not take you out of your window of tolerance. If this happens, it will disrupt your progress in your trauma work or embodied movement practice.

Identifying the edge between activation and over-stimulation is a learning process, but some easy-to-spot signs are a sudden increase or decrease in body temperature, a feeling that you are stuck and cannot move, fogginess, or heightened sensitivity. We don't override warning signals and push spots in our body that resist being engaged within training. But if conditions allow it, we may spend just a moment on the edge between feeling and numbing, seeing if it shifts and observing what comes up. This might be a feeling or a physiological effect, or perhaps an image. Oftentimes a meaningful connection is made.

TAKE ACTION
Establish a Mind-Body Connection
During Warm-up

You may not know which of your muscles, if any, are prone to being offline. That's okay. Doing exercises to intentionally activate your muscles prepares you for a workout generally, as well as helping you acknowledge the state of your different muscle groups as separate from any training plan. For this Take Action, I've provided a series of four isometric hold exercises, in which you contract certain muscles and hold for the duration. I'll walk you through getting into position and specify which body part you should bring your attention to as you hold the form. Simply bringing the intention to foster a connection to this exercise can prepare you to foster a mind-body connection, too.

If you find any of these exercises triggering, stop, and consider using the passing-back-and-forth exercise laid out in the Take Action in Chapter One (on page 32) to self-regulate.

While the exercises listed here are used to activate certain muscles, they're not the only activation exercises out there. If you find these exercises don't work for you for any reason, you may want to do some research into alternatives, or consult with a Corrective Exercise Specialist or physical therapist to find the best ones for you.

I recommend that you try all of these exercises at least once. If you notice that you can't feel a certain muscle as you run through them, there's no cause for alarm—this is just information. Note it down and plan to include that exercise in your regular warm-up with the goal of establishing that connection. In addition, if you have chronic joint pain, you may find that warming up the muscles around that joint will enable you to work out with less pain.

With each exercise, I also include a step for tracking your progress in a training journal. It can be hard to feel like you're seeing progress when that progress is incremental and not always linear, or even just to remember what you did last time. Keeping a record solves both of these issues, as you can easily see what you did each step of the way and just how far you've come.

I also invite you to write down any thoughts or feelings that may come up as you do this work. These exercises are intended to open a dialogue between you and your body, and journaling can be of great help with this, as it allows you to reflect on mental and emotional themes that come up in particular areas. Through this, you can identify which parts may need more encouragement to start to work so you can move efficiently and safely. I suggest you consider bringing up anything you discover that feels important emotionally to a counselor or therapist.

WHAT YOU WILL NEED:
A stopwatch
A mat or comfortable place you can lie on the floor
A towel or washcloth
A chair, bench, or counter (if you need to modify the push-up)
A wall
Your training journal

DURATION:
15 minutes, 2 to 3 times a week

To be done as a warm-up. Additional rounds can be added to form a standalone isometric workout. Each additional round, with rests, will take about 10 minutes.

SPLIT SQUAT ISOMETRIC HOLD

This exercise works with one side of your body at a time, giving you the opportunity to get in touch with both your left and right-lower body.

1. Stand with one side of your body near a wall. This exercise challenges your balance and a wall is an excellent support to have close by, either to catch yourself on or to reach out a hand and steady yourself with as you execute the movement. Keep the free hand—or both if you feel balanced enough—on your hips.
2. Stand with your feet hip distance apart and step one leg forward into a moderately wide split stance (finding the right distance for your feet based on your proportions will take a little exploration). Your front toes should be pointed forward. Allow the heel of your back foot to come up so you're standing on the ball of your foot. It doesn't matter whether you put your right or left foot forward first, as you'll do this on both sides.
3. Keep your front knee forward, in line with your second toe, and envision lowering your torso straight down. Keep your hips pointing forward as you lower yourself. Your front knee will bend, moving forward over your front foot (keep the knee tracking over that second toe), and your back knee will move straight down. Lower yourself just enough that you feel holding the position will be hard, but manageable.
4. Notice your thighs. You should feel the front thigh doing most of the work to maintain this position.
5. Maintain this position for thirty seconds to one minute. If you cannot get to thirty seconds at first, then come up as needed, reset, and work toward this duration in as few rounds as possible.

6. To come out of this position, imagine pushing yourself away from the floor and follow through by extending your legs, then step your feet together.
7. Repeat, stepping the opposite leg forward.
8. Take a moment to note how long you held the position, what you felt, and where you felt it, in your journal. As always, you're encouraged to include any other thoughts or feelings that come up as you do this exercise.

GLUTE BRIDGE ISOMETRIC HOLD

You'll do this exercise in order to establish a connection with your body's largest, often most underused muscles—your gluteal muscles, or glutes (also known as your bum). In this exercise, you want to initiate the movement from your glutes. As you do it, if you feel that the back of your thighs are doing most of the work, bring your heels closer to your bum.

1. Lie on your back with your knees bent and the soles of your feet on the floor, hip distance apart.
2. Squeeze your glute muscles as if you're trying to keep from passing gas.
3. Maintaining the hold, slowly scoop your pelvis up (it should be a small movement) and then lift your bum straight up, as high as you can, while ensuring the movement comes from squeezing your glutes. Try to not dip into your back or arch into a backbend and avoid pushing your hips up with momentum, because this will lead you to primarily use other muscles to come up.
4. Once you get to your maximum lift (this may only be an inch or two, or it may be that your hips are fully extended, creating a straight line from knee to waist) maintain that hold, squeezing for thirty seconds to one minute. If you cannot get to thirty seconds at first, then come down as needed, reset, and work toward this duration in as few rounds as possible.

5. As you squeeze, check in with how your knees are doing. They should remain pointed to the ceiling, not turning in or out.

6. To come out of this form, lower your hips in a slow, controlled way.

7. Each week increase your hold time by fifteen seconds, until you can hold for ninety seconds.

8. Take a moment to note how long you held the position, what you felt, and where you felt it, in your journal. As always, you're encouraged to include any other thoughts or feelings that come up as you do this exercise.

PUSH-UP ISOMETRIC HOLD

Traditional push-ups are hard to do, but there are easy ways to modify them to meet your ability level. For this exercise, you may want to start with your hands on the wall or a kitchen counter and push against that. You can make this movement more challenging as needed by gradually getting your body into a more horizontal position. If pushing against the wall feels too easy, try placing your hands on the seat of a chair, coffee table or other low object and push against that, eventually working your way to pushing yourself up from the floor itself. This exercise works a number of muscles in the trunk of your body, but here we're primarily getting in touch with the chest muscles.

As a modification for sensitive wrists, make your hands into fists with knuckles against the floor or other support, holding your wrists straight while you execute the movement.

1. If you're using a wall, stand facing the wall at arm's length. Reach forward and place your palms (or fists) against it, slightly wider than the width of your shoulders. If you're using a counter, stand facing the counter and place your palms (or fists) along its edge. For any lower surfaces, including the floor, place your hands down slightly more than shoulder width apart, and with straight arms and legs, come up into a plank position on the balls of your feet.

2. Bend your elbows out slightly to the side and lower your whole body. To keep your body in a straight line, squeeze your glutes and abs. Your elbows should bend and your upper arm should make a 45-degree angle (or less) with your body. If you feel this exercise primarily in your shoulders, bring your hands closer together.

3. Once you've bent your elbows 90 degrees so that you're halfway down, maintain the position for at least fifteen seconds and up to one minute. If you cannot get to fifteen seconds at first, then come up as needed, reset, and work toward this duration in as few rounds as possible.

4. Notice what you feel in your chest.

5. To come out of this position from the wall, push yourself upright. To raise yourself from a lower height, push yourself upright and then bring your feet or knees together one at a time underneath you. If you're doing this on the floor, lower your knees to help you come upright.

6. Take a moment to note how long you held the position, what you felt, and where you felt it, in your journal. As always, you're encouraged to include any other thoughts or feelings that come up as you do this exercise.

LYING Y-RAISE ISOMETRIC HOLD

Last, but never least, you're going to get in touch with the muscles of your upper back through the following exercise.

1. Place a rolled-up washcloth or towel toward the top of your mat. Lie on it face-down, forehead on the towel, with your arms extended overhead so your body creates a Y-shape. Check that your elbows are straight and thumbs are pointed up in the air.

2. Squeeze the muscles around your shoulder blades. It should feel like you're pulling your shoulder blades down and back slightly, as if you were trying to slide them into your back pockets, and should cause your arms to lift up an inch or so. Avoid squeezing your neck muscles or bringing your shoulders up to your ears.

3. Keeping your arms straight, hold this position for fifteen seconds to one minute. As you contract the muscles of your upper back, try to feel them working.
4. Lower your arms in a slow, controlled way.
5. Take a moment to note how long you held the position, what you felt, and where you felt it, in your journal. As always, you're encouraged to include any other thoughts or feelings that come up as you do this exercise.

CHAPTER SIX
Trauma and Time

TRAUMA MAKES US TIME TRAVELERS—but not in a cool, adventurous way, like in the movies *Back to The Future* or *Bill and Ted's Excellent Adventure*. Our experiences time traveling through trauma are dark, surreal, and far from "excellent." We are not in control of our time machines: trauma is. Our time machines don't look like cool cars with hydraulic doors or tricked-out phone booths, but are something more complex, yet also ordinary: our own bodies. Irrespective of our personal narrative, trauma lingers, ready to transport us from the present moment to the past incident by way of triggers, intrusive memories, old sensations, and flashbacks. As far as your nervous system is concerned, unprocessed trauma, whether remembered or not, is not entirely in your past. It remains with you even now, unmoored from time. It takes up residence in your body, causing you to repeat patterns of movement, phrases, behavior, and meaning-making, revealing that you haven't yet processed what happened and left it in the past.

The good news is that we *can* process traumatic events after the fact and anchor them in our timeline, in the past, where they belong. At this point, they're integrated into our narrative as opposed to interfering with it. This is intense work, but I have done it and have seen others do it, and I believe that you can do it, too (otherwise I wouldn't have written this book!).

It was in 2018, during my first Somatic Experiencing (SE) training module, when I grasped that, although our physical self doesn't always understand that a trauma is over, we can teach our nervous system that it is. SE employs a series of tools to help you process your trauma and come to understand on a deep, neurological level that the trauma is over, and that you have survived. Once your body understands that, you can move from surviving to thriving. I integrate SE practices and models into my work and my daily life, and have found great success with it.

WHY I LOVE SOMATIC EXPERIENCING FOR TRAUMA WORK

Somatic Experiencing is a body-oriented approach to healing trauma and stress disorders. I first learned of it when I began to research whether emotional trauma could, in fact, be causing the tremendous back pain that sometimes left me bedbound. The Somatic Experiencing Trauma Institute describes SE on its website as the product of Dr. Peter Levine's "lifelong study of stress physiology, psychology, ethology, biology, neuroscience, indigenous healing practices, and medical biophysics."[1] It's an interdisciplinary approach that focuses not only on the thoughts and emotions that come up in trauma treatment, but also on bodily responses like sensations and behaviors. I like the way it recognizes that our bodies are composed of numerous interconnected systems working as a whole, and that our thoughts, emotions, sensations, and behaviors all contain vital information and impact one another.

I also love that SE works by giving us the time and space to process unprocessed trauma. If we're unable to complete the trauma response to flee, fight, or otherwise save ourselves in the moment of a traumatic event because we were thwarted, trapped, or stuck, our nervous systems will often also stay stuck there, reenacting the trauma response far into the future through our behaviors (i.e., panic attacks, collapsing) or our relationships.

Have you had the experience of recounting a story of something horrible that happened to you, and your body started to feel just like it did in that moment, as if you were back there? Maybe you got all speedy in your narration and your body tightened. Or maybe you were very detached, barely emoting, even though it's a harrowing story. The telling of a story like this is usually a visceral experience, even if we don't realize it. This can leave you feeling lousy, because you're reliving something awful that you haven't yet processed on a physiological level.

Although traumas can be narrowed down to a point in time, examined closely, and securely placed in the past, they cannot be untangled from the fabric of our lives. They cannot be erased. All we can do is understand, on both a physical and emotional level, that we are no longer in that traumatizing situation. Once trauma is secured in the past, it no longer directs our lives. It becomes just one part of our much larger story. It is integrated, but never gone.

SE allows your physical self to join you in the present moment, as opposed to being stuck in the past moment of trauma. And a Somatic Experiencing Practitioner (SEP) is like a thought, feeling, and time travel-guide who accompanies you on your journey. Through talk, movement, and occasionally light touch, SEPs support clients as they experience sensations, images, effects, and realizations while recounting moments around trauma. Like many other strategies for healing from trauma, this is done slowly and rarely by going straight for the trauma moment, instead arriving at it after exploring the surrounding moments.

SOMATIC EXPERIENCING IN PRACTICE

My therapist uses SE techniques and tools with me. These helped me heal even when I was erratically time traveling and feeling completely unhinged, uncertain of what would trigger me and when. Together, we were able to steadily make progress using a combination of SE and other tools, so that, as with titration, my physiology was able to tolerate more and more stress and I could begin to unpack my heavy emotional baggage.

I don't know about you, but when I find something to be profoundly helpful, I want to know all about it, understand the way it works, and then share this information with everyone else. And as I found SE to be profoundly helpful, I am now in training to be an SEP myself.

During my first training module, I gathered with about sixty students to watch a recording of SE's founder, Dr. Levine, working with a man named Ray in 2008.[2] Ray had served as a Marine in Iraq and Afghanistan and was almost killed by two IEDs. He woke up two weeks after the incident in hospital, unable to walk or talk. Although he eventually regained these functions, his quality of life was severely diminished. He was diagnosed with traumatic brain injury (TBI), severe PTSD, chronic pain, depression, and Tourette's Syndrome. Ray was on several medications, couldn't deal with people, and would not even look up at Dr. Levine when they began their work together.

I invite you to pause and check in with yourself.
Perhaps you can allow yourself to sense that you are
supported by the seat, bed, or ground below you.

The video is edited to show Ray's progress over several sessions. In the first session, we witness him beginning to move out of shock, becoming more present in the current time and starting to acknowledge that the IEDs detonated in the past, rather than feeling like he was still immersed in the experience. None of us can process an overwhelming event if we feel like we are still living it. It took four sessions to move through this initial stage and allow Ray to go deeper, to explore the feelings below the shock.

Levine reported that during the fifth session, they began to go deeper into Ray's feelings of losing his friends when the IED detonated. It was in the video of this fifth session that his Tourette's symptoms seemed to abate somewhat, and there was a greater calmness visible in him. He was embodied and could feel things—like a shaking deep inside himself. Dr. Levine invited Ray to say the following words: "I'm alive. I'm alive and I'm here." Ray repeated the words while staying embodied, and Dr. Levine asked him what he felt. "Rage. Sorrow. Anger."

This is a famous video within the SE community. Watching it that first time, I found Ray relatable and honest. I love the way he admits in a later interview that when he first started to work with Dr. Levine, he thought what they were doing "was the dumbest thing in the world." But he also admits that once their work started, he began to think, "What if this work can really make me better? What if I (was) stopping myself from getting better? You know what? Screw this. Let's put forth the energy needed to make this work and get better." I found his candor very refreshing. Ray first looked at his pile of heavy things and thought, "This is stupid," but he began to lift them anyway and started to notice that it was actually helping.

But I don't think this was the most poignant takeaway. For me, it was that statement in the fifth session where Ray acknowledged out loud that he had survived, and that he was alive.

Watching the video in my training session, I stood in the back of the room and rocked from left to right, regulating myself. Tears streamed uncontrollably down my face. I slowed down my movement and lowered myself to sit on the floor. Although the group was around me, they faded from my awareness. The video played on. As I wept, Ray continued to repeat to Dr. Levine, "I survived. Not everyone did. And I'm here. And I'm alive."

I suppose Ray was processing survivor's guilt, which in his case manifested as Tourette's Syndrome and depression. I was processing grief, which had been showing up as hypervigilance, anxiety, and rigidity. In that moment, I realized that perhaps I had never told myself "I survived" in a manner that my nervous system could understand. While I would enthusiastically share the story of watching the Ray video with friends who listened, I never shared my sneaking suspicion that I still didn't quite understand, deep in my bones, that *I was alive.* That I had survived and my trauma was in the past. How much time had I lost by not truly understanding that my trauma was over?

FEELING FREEDOM FROM SOMATIC EXPERIENCING

A few months after I watched the Ray video, I was sitting in my therapist's neutral yet modern office, in my usual spot on her firm leather sofa. Many of our sessions now blend together, as if they were one sea of emotion and meaning-making, but there are some sessions that stand out like buoys on the water's surface. It was during these that I experienced not just some greater understanding of my world, but a complete paradigm shift. This session was one of those. It only took four words. First, my therapist said, "I am going to invite you to say something."

I braced myself. My stomach suddenly felt as if the bottom had dropped out, leaving behind the dull ache I associate with dread. As an SEP-in-training, I knew what was coming. You know that moment when you know what someone's about to say and you don't want them to? A television drama would have used slow motion to capture my body registering it: a sideways glance, a hard swallow, and a visible readying for impact. We would know that the protagonist—in this case, me—was afraid.

Then my therapist said, "I am going to invite you to say, 'I survived. I'm alive.'"

With a suddenly dry mouth, I turned my gaze away from her direction and toward the window. I was looking at nothing in particular.

"I survived," I said, just above a whisper. Although I was sitting rather still, my lurching insides suddenly ground to a halt. It was as if, on the inside, I had been running for my life as fast as I could, and reality had finally caught up with me, grabbed me, and said, "STOP! It's over."

My eyes dropped and my head swiveled back toward my therapist, but I didn't look at her. My gaze was pointed at the rug by her feet, but I wasn't looking at the rug. I was looking inward—time-traveling back to the present, leaving the past in its place. Had I been running for years?

"I am alive," I continued, this time a little louder. My breath returned and my body found calm and stillness. I wept, but it was gentle, not heaving sobs. It wasn't catharsis; it was a pause that was allowing my body to catch up with my lived experience. I had survived. I was alive. My body finally understood that what had happened was in the past.

I invite you to pause and check in with yourself.
Consider standing up, stretching and
maybe having a sip of water.

Unlike Ray, I didn't repeat this step multiple times. Once was enough for that moment. There was no feeling of advancing the narrative, or of meaning-making, when I was done. Where my thoughts normally resided, there was instead a quiet spaciousness. Throughout my trunk, arms, and legs, there was an internal sensation of quick, light movement—like lots of tiny ballerinas assuming new positions across the stage inside my body. "Change of plans," my internal choreographer-nervous system declared: "We are done running. Everyone, pirouette or leap to your new stations." And everyone obliged, flying lightly and gracefully but with speed to their new spots in my internal world. I just had to wait a bit for them to land and once there, they could rest. Was this my system reorganizing itself?

It took me a long time to arrive at this point, where I could place at least one trauma firmly in the timeline of my past, and my body could finally understand that it was over. When my thoughts came back online, my first one was, "Holy shit.". I have no memory of what transpired immediately after that. All I remember is knowing that something very profound had just happened. I probably went straight home and took a nap.

Realizing that I was alive and the threat was gone set the stage for me to really engage with life again. It allowed me to complete my body's natural threat response, process the original trauma, and minimize instances of sudden time traveling. Although my symptoms had lessened in the months immediately following my trauma, I had not yet healed. Parts of me didn't understand that it was safe to move on, so I was still spending a tremendous amount of energy on living like I was under threat. Once I explicitly worked to show my body that it was okay, I felt safe to unfurl and flourish again, like I had a few years prior when I took up barbell sports. I was free to step into my aliveness once more.

I had one client with whom I did Somatic Experiencing work around an experience with a previous personal trainer, who had unwittingly overwhelmed and triggered her during multiple sessions. She didn't want to go back to her trainer, quite understandably, but she was also afraid of it happening again with someone new, and she began to feel as if she couldn't even set foot into a gym without panicking.

We had a couple of priorities. The first was to come up with a workout strategy that would support and teach her how to identify her own boundaries in the gym, as well as giving her the practical tools to enforce them. Then we'd use SE to process the incidents with the past trainer that were preventing her from coming back to the gym now, despite wanting to. She had a narrative around the trigger but chose not to share it with me, so I worked with her experience with the trainer instead.

After taking the time to make sure the environment felt good to her, identifying her resources, and building a rapport, I asked her to describe a typical day when she was seeing this trainer, starting with getting up in the morning. Her morning routine included breakfast, getting dressed, and tending to her family. There was rhythm in her voice and natural movement in her body as she spoke, until she said: "Then I get in the car with my husband to go to the gym."

Responding to a hard swallow and the sudden stiffness in her body language, I jumped in before she could continue and said, "Okay, I'm going to stop you there and invite you to pause and check in with yourself. Are there any sensations, thoughts, or images coming up for you when you mention getting in the car with your husband to go to the gym?"

I was interrupting her story to give her the opportunity to notice and process the information in her body. It's one of the techniques of SE—sometimes maddening, yet very effective therapeutically—for an SEP to continually interrupt. This isn't to simply change the subject, like a rude uncle who can't wait to hear his own voice; they interrupt you to slow you down, so that you can fully take in the experience you're recounting. The interruptions add pockets of time to cushion the overwhelming moments, making it easier for you to finish processing your thwarted defensive response.

"Um. Um, yes," my client answered my question. "I feel a shaking rising in my . . ." She tapped her sternum to indicate where she felt it.

"Okay. Would it feel okay to stay with that sensation for a bit?" I asked, wanting not to overwhelm her but to give her the opportunity to process her activation.

"Yes. That would be okay," she replied. We spent some time tracking this sensation. Every so often, I would ask her to move to more neutral spots in her body. By directing the conversation, stopping frequently and shifting gears, I helped her move toward the edge of her window of tolerance and then back into the safe middle. I want to note that we didn't get past this part of the narrative during the session—we stayed in the car. After a few minutes, she let out a deep breath through her nose and her body softened. We closed the session there. Over the course of several more, we were able to process what had happened with her previous trainer and eventually, she felt free to pursue other fitness modalities. And although we never had an "I am alive" moment together, she did feel empowered to return to the gym and train, which showed me that she was beginning to take control of her timeline and anchor these incidents in the past.

TAKE ACTION
Settle and Integrate

Processing trauma is heavy lifting and it can provoke moments of nervous system arousal. After spending time and energy processing a piece of your trauma, no matter the modality you use, I strongly urge you to take a moment to settle your system, find some calm, and make space to integrate the work you've done before moving on. In this exercise, I'll describe a self-care practice that uses touch through placing your own hands on your head, neck, shoulders, and trunk.

WHAT YOU WILL NEED:
Clothing that allows easy access to your arms and hands
A place where you won't be disturbed

DURATION:
3 to 4 minutes

1. Take a moment to feel yourself being supported by your seat or the floor beneath you. If you'd like, take a breath, inhaling and exhaling through your nose. You will now move through a sequence of hand-to-body positions. Spend twenty to thirty seconds in each, or however long feels right to you.

2. Close your eyes and, with your palms to your face, fingers pointing up, place the heels of your hands on your eyes or cheekbones (whichever feels better) and let your fingers rest on your forehead.

3. Next, with your eyes open or closed, cup the center of your forehead with one hand while cradling the back of your head with the other, applying equal amounts of gentle pressure. Let your fingers point wherever feels natural.

4. For the third position, bring your hands to your shoulders, either by crossing your arms over your chest and placing your hands on opposite shoulders, or by placing each hand on its respective shoulder and lowering your elbows. Apply gentle downward pressure.

5. Next, bring your hands to your back, near your waist if possible, and support the back of your body.

6. For the final position, bring one hand to your forehead and the other to the center of your chest, providing support to the front of your body.

7. End with your hands in an easy position, perhaps prayer, with your chin somewhat tucked. Feel for either your breath on your fingertips or sensations in and around your hands. Thank yourself for taking this moment to provide yourself with support and care.

CHAPTER SEVEN

Strength Training as an Embodied Movement Practice

I N CASE YOU HAVEN'T REALIZED IT YET, I'm more than just a barbell-loving meathead. My movement story has had interludes of an on-again, off-again yoga practice that started years before I began lifting weights. The first time I took a yoga class was in 1998, when I registered for it in college to fulfill the PE requirement I resented with every fiber of my being. Although I'm proud to be part of a tradition of women's education and believe that women are as strong as men, I was really annoyed that our school's founder, Mary Lyon, valued exercise so much that one hundred and sixty years after the school's founding—and after a lifetime of traumatic gym classes for me—I was still required to take four terms of physical education. There were plenty of options, but yoga sounded like the easiest and least-offensive one to my gym-hating self. "I could stretch for an hour," I thought to myself. I didn't understand then that yoga is much more than stretching.

Despite its 6:30 a.m. start time, yoga was a popular class (clearly, I wasn't the only undergrad who had the same thought about stretching). The teacher, Donna, was a kind yet no-nonsense fitness professional with a sensible haircut. I would show up bleary eyed, often just four hours after I'd gone to bed, and find a spot among the other forty-odd sleepy young women to unroll my school-issued yoga mat, the thwacking of the rubber hitting the floor becoming a signal to my system that mandated movement was about to begin. We would start seated and move through a familiar sequence of sun salutations, which I always despised because I was certain Downward Dog could only lead to unfortunate embarrassment at best. On top of that, when I did the pose, my wrists and shoulders hurt and my sweaty hands and feet would slide on my mat, threatening a belly-flop. I could just imagine a loud thud, followed by my own small "Ow! Ugh, I'm okay," interrupting everyone else's meditative moment. I was ashamed of how much I was sweating in a "stretching class." For the first four or five classes, I felt like that little girl in her elementary school gym who desperately wanted to disappear.

One morning, before class started, I went over to Donna and told her I had to talk to her. I felt awful; I was exhausted, stressed out from midterm exams, and had horrendous menstrual cramps. She was tough but also approachable and kind. She looked me in the eye while she listened. She thought for a moment and then set me up—lying on my back, on a bolster cushion centered along the length of my mat, with my legs bent and rotated outward at the hips, the soles of my feet touching. She placed blocks under my knees and suggested I let my arms rest out to my sides.

"You can stay like this for the whole class," Donna said matter-of-factly, then walked away.

Really? Uh, okay, I thought to myself, since her quick departure left me unable to respond.

After just a few seconds in the position, I thought, *Hmm. This is kind of nice.* What if yoga could be something I might like?

Grateful to have Donna's approval to lie down, and for the support of the yoga equipment holding my body, I stayed in Reclined Bound Angle Pose until the end of class, when I shifted into Savasana with everyone else by removing the bolster and blocks, then lying on my back with my legs extended and arms resting naturally at my sides. That day, I fell in love with Reclined Bound Angle Pose, and I still do it today to chill myself out.

Over time during that semester, I started finding yoga enjoyable—even the more challenging bits. Restorative poses like Supported Reclined Bound Angle really helped me feel grounded and at ease, and with some corrections (and a lot of practice) I felt more comfortable in poses like Downward Dog, too. Although it was enjoyable, the way I was practicing yoga then was not embodied. For yoga or any other practice to be embodied, you have to focus your awareness on the sensations in your body brought on by the exercise. The only intention I was bringing was to pass the class.

BEYOND YOGA: THE WORLD OF EMBODIED MOVEMENT

Embodied movement is a movement-based mindfulness practice. Yoga, along with qigong, the Feldenkrais Method, and the Alexander Technique, are a few practices that commonly fall into this category, but an embodied approach can be applied to any sort of movement. If you're staying present while you wiggle your fingers, dig in the dirt, twirl around your living room, or lift heavy things, then you are engaging in embodied movement.

I think there are common misconceptions about all sorts of movement practices. That lifting weights is for getting rid of angry energy, and yoga is an easy solution to pain and stress, are the two I perhaps encounter the most. From my experience, I know that yoga isn't always easy or harmless, and that lifting weights can be a grounding meditation.

Qigong, the Feldenkrais Method, the Alexander Technique, and certain types of yoga are explicitly referred to as embodied movement practices. This is because, when done as intended, the person practicing them pays attention to their interoceptive experience, or what it feels like in their body as they move. They may also tune in to their proprioception, which is the sense of where their body is as it moves through space, and kinesthetics, which is the way their body is moving. There is growing interest among the scientific community in the ways embodied movement practices can support physical health and wellness; some studies have found that they can alleviate the symptoms of a number of health issues, including chronic pain, and mental health issues like anxiety and depression.[1]

Even though there are many options, yoga tends to be the western go-to for embodied movement practice. Even back in 1998, I knew I was supposed to find it relaxing, even though I had no idea why. In 2018, thirty-six million Americans reported practicing yoga and over six thousand yoga studios were open to welcome them. Nearly a third of all Americans try yoga at some point, and many do so specifically to find stress relief.[2] When the COVID-19 pandemic closed studios, there seemed to be a surge of people taking virtual yoga classes online. According to Mindbody, a wellness class and services app, twenty percent of active users reported booking an online yoga class in 2019, but by June 2020 this was up to about eighty percent of active users.[3]

Given all this, it doesn't surprise me that when a doctor or therapist suggests embodied movement as a healing practice, we might be inclined to turn to the nearest yoga studio or most popular online yoga class. I know I have. And with the growing interest in developing trauma therapies, there are ever-increasing options for trauma-informed yoga programs for people looking for an embodied movement practice.

Personally, I've found yoga to be helpful at times—with chronic pain, anxiety, and depression, like studies suggest—but as with anything in life, it's not the right solution for everyone. In fact, it wasn't always the right solution for me. Over the years, both before [   ] and after, my yoga practice ebbed and flowed in its regularity. I think that's pretty normal. There's something you love to do and at times you do it daily, while at others you don't get to spend as much time doing it, but you always come back. I know people who have this relationship with their art, gardening, various sports, and other hobbies.

Before I developed PTSD, Slow Flow Vinyasa yoga was a great help in mitigating my symptoms of depression, anxiety, and back pain. But after I developed PTSD, any form of yoga, even if taught by someone with training in trauma-sensitive yoga, would trigger in me excessive arousal and flashbacks.

When I moved back to New York City in 2006, I found a yoga studio that I loved four blocks from my apartment. However, by 2014, I had all but dropped it for strength training. As good as yoga felt, strength training did more for my back and made me feel more alive and powerful, like Mountain Pose but amplified a thousand times. But at the end of 2014, I had to take a break from barbells, dumbbells, and kettlebells because I sustained a back injury so severe that it left me bedridden for weeks and took over a year to recover from.

When I developed PTSD in early 2014, my symptoms gave birth to many new, extreme behaviors. For example, I wouldn't watch any television at all. Now that might not seem extreme to some people, but there were points in my past when I'd been struggling with my mental health and all I did was watch TV. Not only did I now refuse to watch it; I was actually angry that so many other people watched it while completely unaware of how it could be harmful to others, like myself. This PTSD symptom, known as avoidant behavior, also kept me from walking down certain streets, being in certain places, and from consuming a lot of media for fear of being triggered.

Another symptom I suffered from was hyperarousal. I was easily startled and always on the lookout for danger. Hyperarousal contributed to what would become a compulsive approach to strength training. I'd begun the practice eight years prior, doing at most four days a week, purely to take care of myself. With PTSD though, it morphed into a daily regimen of pushing myself as hard as possible, as if I was preparing for battle.

I coupled compulsive training with my old coping mechanism of dissociating from pain. Dissociation had gotten me through my previous emotional pain and bouts of chronic back pain. I pushed through discomfort and injury. People can do this for pretty long periods of time—I did it for about six weeks. If you follow professional sports, you frequently see the great human ability to override pain signals in action. A quarterback may injure his elbow or shoulder mid-season, but he plays through the whole season and then gets joint surgery later. A professional athlete usually plays through pain, at least in part, because millions of dollars and his job are on the line. Also, the rest of his life is set up to help him recover.

But I'm not a professional athlete. I am a person who is an average performer at sports that you cannot go pro in. And, probably like you, my life is not set up so I can spend the entire off-season recovering. (There's no off-season in the sport of being human!) I don't make any money based on my sports performance—in fact, training costs me money. And most folks cannot afford the cost or time for surgery or rehab. Most people in the world, and in the gym, are not professional athletes, so it's unhealthy for them to train like they are. But even so, every day, I would show up at the gym and aggressively lift as much as I could, stressing out my body and ignoring how it felt. This way of training is in opposition to what I now know to be good for long-term health and resilience. No one at the gym pulled me aside to ask, "Why are you training like this?" In fact, quite the contrary: my work ethic, discipline, and drive to become unstoppable were celebrated. The only person who asked was my therapist.

"I want to be as strong as possible," I said.

"Why do you want to be as strong as possible?"

"So . . . I am ready for . . . anything," I replied in a stilted manner. Even talking about my fear of being harmed scared me and, to be honest, I hadn't given much thought to my compulsion for getting stronger. I was trying to keep it together as intrusive images flashed in my mind's eye.

"What might 'anything' be?" she volleyed back to me.

At this question, I thought *she* was crazy, which is an unsettling thought to have about your own therapist. My eyes darted right to the door. I didn't feel like staying, but I didn't feel like going either. As far as I was concerned, threats loomed just over my shoulder and around every corner, and I felt that I had to be prepared to face this seemingly inevitable threat. This conversation was years before the story from Chapter Six, when I sat across from her and realized I was alive. This was before we used Somatic Experiencing at all. I trusted her and knew she had many wonderful insights, but I wasn't yet confident that she understood how I experienced the world.

In fact, I believed that I wasn't doing *enough* to be strong. I was doing Olympic weightlifting and had taken up karate prior to [   ], so to become even stronger, I took up a third sport: powerlifting. I trained in powerlifting three days a week. I continued Olympic lifting two days a week and I was also taking karate five days a week. There are only seven days in a week, people! So I was training ten times a week, enabled by the "CRUSH IT! BEAST MODE!" mentality of many of the fitness professionals around me. Even if you aren't a gym-goer, you might recognize this messaging from your social media feed: your cousin/high school friend/co-worker/ex-lover posts images of muscular bodies dripping with sweat, chalk on their hands, a look of determination on their face as if this were a battle to the death, and all-caps text declaring "NO EXCUSES!"

BEYOND PAIN: ACKNOWLEDGING LIMITS WITH EMBODIED MOVEMENT

By now, I bet you can recognize a pattern here. It was during the aforementioned therapy session that I began to see it, too. Some small part of me recognized that my training was compulsive and that, just maybe, living as if threats were lurking around every corner was not "normal." But I was at a total loss as to how to stop it and had limited self-compassion, so I just kept going to the gym and the dojo and doing double training days.

By the time I became aware of this dissonance, I hated myself. I hated how I was living my life. I hated that I was living in fear all the time. My compulsive lifting was an attempt at not constantly living in fear, but I was instead having more flashbacks, as I was making myself more susceptible to them by training so hard and so often. I repeatedly pushed myself out of my window of tolerance and rarely rested. It wasn't just that my mind was frightened and angry—my whole body was.

It was also starting to hurt again. My back was threatening to go out. When I reracked the bar after a squat or a bench press and moved to stand upright, it would seize for a moment, just like that day in college. If I moved slowly enough then I could stand all the way up. As the weeks progressed, each step sent an ever-growing tingle that started from my bum and worked its way down my leg. Sometimes I would wince but I would always keep going. Training was a compulsion, not a passion, and with that mindset, when my back began to bother me I decided the best solution was to ignore the pain in order to train more. The thinking was that if I could lift more weight, I would be stronger and my back would be okay.

Surprise! I was wrong. Instead, I completely leveled myself. My back pain had returned and, just like everything else my body was doing, it was extreme. On November 1, 2014, I woke up with sciatica so severe that I experienced partial paralysis in my left leg. My back was spasming so hard that any small movement was an excruciating challenge. I was barely able to get out of bed. I was thirty-six years old.

I thought I'd been scared before, but being this immobilized was completely terrifying. I realized that I could no longer run and fight. I found my rock bottom and was left to my own devices to figure out how to actually take care of my body.

It took months of physical therapy before I could do much more with my body than make it to PT and therapy. For weeks, I only did simple supported exercises and received soft tissue work. I was frustrated and angry with these limitations, which made me afraid I'd lost the body I had convinced myself was strong and worthy, and which others now praised in ways I'd never previously experienced. I certainly couldn't lift weights, but I was desperate to find another movement practice to do as I recovered. So, I looked to my old standby: yoga.

Over the years, I learned that yoga could be practiced in a way that meets you where you are on any given day—like on that day in 1998, when I lay on the floor while my classmates hit Downward Dog again and again. I decided the trick was to find the right teacher and a studio that would honor this way of practicing.

I tried various classes at different studios and even trauma-informed private instruction, but I consistently found that yoga triggered hyperarousal and back pain. No matter what, it felt unsafe, so having learned my lesson the hard way, I honored my body and crossed yoga off my list. I didn't know why it was so triggering at the time, and it felt too dangerous to stick around to figure it out. Later on, I learned this was the same feeling of overwhelm that Dr. Gallagher had described; I was going from dissociated to completely over-stimulated, like my client with the shoulder and back pain. Just getting in touch with the unprocessed excess of arousal still in my system was too much. Instead, I got my creative juices flowing and decided to combine two of my resources: my love of lifting and my knack for research. I was determined to figure out how to get back into the gym. And I did.

It took time, effort, research, and practice, but eventually I felt safe enough to get back under the barbell. It was a year before I could do strength training outside of physical therapy and longer than that before I could practice strength sports. During that time, I came to realize that I could only ensure proper form if I stayed present with every repetition and honored my body's signals when I was approaching the edge of my window of tolerance. At some point, I realized that even though I was engaging in something not commonly recognized as a mindful movement practice, I actually was engaging in embodied movement. Embodied movement is always mindful of the body and its sensations—so much so, that I think of embodied and mindful movement as one and the same.

An easy way to understand mindfulness is to think of an activity with an anchor or object of focus. In seated mindfulness, or meditation, the object of focus is often the breath. The practitioner is instructed to "stay with" or "observe" their breath. What makes movement mindful isn't the movement itself, but where you put your attention as you do the movement. The object of your focus then is interoception—what it feels like in your body as you engage in practice. Staying with that object mentally makes the practice mindful and inherently embodied.

Doing something without mindfulness, on the other hand, might look like wiggling your fingers while you think about what you're going to eat for lunch, or doing a bicep curl as you plan your next #flexfriday social media post instead of really experiencing using your bicep muscle to bend your arm at the elbow.

Mindfulness is just one part of an embodied movement practice, though. There is also the *practice* part, which comes into play whenever your attention inevitably shifts away from the object of focus. Yes, I said inevitably, because your attention *will* waver. This isn't because something is wrong with you. It is just part of being a person. Believe it or not, even mindfulness teachers experience wandering thoughts. Their practice is the same as yours. It requires acknowledging that your focus has shifted and, compassionately and without judgment, coming back to the object of your focus: in this case, what it feels like to move within your body. The non-judgmental and compassionate part is important. When your attention shifts, it's an opportunity to practice noticing this and coming back to your body. It's not a mistake or a failure; it is the practice. You start with an anchor, get distracted, and then come back to it.

I assure you that, despite the simplicity of this guideline, cultivating a mindful movement practice is a challenge. It is also very much worth the work. Through it, you not only take care of yourself from workout to workout by being careful to move correctly and with your lid flipped on, but also set yourself up to act in ways that are healing and promote change, even when change is hard. You'll also become equipped to understand and enforce your boundaries even when trauma has breached them, or if you never had healthy boundaries modeled for you before. And crucially, you will give yourself the tools you need to increase your capacity for stress and widen your window of tolerance.

HOW TO MOVE WITH MINDFULNESS

Before we get deeper into how an embodied movement practice supports change and healing, let's talk about setting yourself up to lift weights as an embodied practice. The principle is simple: think about what your body is doing at every moment, instead of what the weight is doing or anything else you could be thinking about. If you've had a fitness coach at all, you may have already heard this advice. Many good coaches know that preparing in a way that supports embodied movement makes a better lifter, even if that's not how they talk about it. Some of the biggest names in barbell sports coaching tell new athletes that their focus should be on what their body is doing, not what they're trying to do with the bar. For example, three-time world-record holding powerlifter and coach Greg Nuckols writes the following in *How to Deadlift: The Definitive Guide*:

> "Beyond gripping the bar and pulling (it) into your body to keep your lats engaged, your focus should not be on the bar itself.
>
> When you focus on moving the bar, it's easier to lose focus on what your body is doing. Generally, when people who are relatively new to the movement think 'pick the bar up,' all the work they put into their setup goes out the window; their hips shoot way up, their back rounds, and they find themselves in a generally shitty (and less safe) position."

Nuckols doesn't call this "embodied movement," but that is exactly what he is describing. The best way to move well is to focus on what your body is doing as you move it. That's it. When I do a deadlift, which involves picking a barbell off the ground and standing up with it while leaving my arms hanging down in front of me, I feel my feet press into the ground and push the ground away, rather than feeling for the bar moving. I stay with the feeling of my feet pressing into the ground for the first repetition of the lift and all repetitions thereafter. Staying in my body keeps me safe, improves my technique, and gives me the opportunity to practice staying with my interoception under the stress of lifting heavy things. It can do the same for you.

After using a warm-up that allows you to feel connected to all of your muscles, you'll want to practice tapping into those connections again and again as you lift heavy things in the gym (and outside it). For every pull and push of the weight, your attention should be on what your muscles are doing, not what the weight is doing or how you look as you lift. The weight and your reflection are outside of you, and to stay embodied, your practice requires that you pay attention to what's going on inside of you.

As you experience fatigue and maybe even some discomfort from lifting heavy things, it may become increasingly hard to stay with the movement. Your thoughts will wander and that's okay, because now's the time to practice—practice coming back to your anchor, which is yourself, even when that's hard. And if it feels too hard to continue, that's okay too. That is an opportunity to practice listening to your own boundaries and stopping, which we will explore in the next two chapters.

TAKE ACTION
Learn to Hip Hinge Mindfully

If I was only allowed to do one movement with a barbell, it would be a deadlift. The deadlift and its variations are an efficient way to build strength, develop trunk stability, and keep you healthy outside of the gym. It also releases a rush of vitality through my system. I like to teach it to people so they can use this movement when they need to cultivate and feel into their resilience, strength, and aliveness.

The deadlift relies on a movement pattern known as the hip hinge. Like the name implies, it's an action that comes from the hip joint— bending down and then straightening back up—as opposed to the vertebrae in your back. When you pick up something small off the floor, like a sock, you likely bend along the spine to form a c-shape and then stand back up. In doing so, you primarily use a series of small muscles in your back. Socks are very light so that's most likely not a problem. But let's say you want to pick up something really heavy. You'd want to use your biggest muscles, your glutes, to do so. I don't care how big or small your bum is—your glutes, the muscles that make it up, are definitely stronger than the long, skinny erector spinae muscles in your back that helped you pick up your sock. When you do a hip hinge correctly, you use your glutes to move and your back stays stable, like a tabletop.

I have taught the hip hinge in workshops, foundations classes, and private sessions, so I've seen all the ways people try to move without being embodied. While it's a simple movement, many of us aren't accustomed to it, so it's not always easy to execute. As such, I'm going to walk you through how to do a proper hip hinge, which is the foundation of many different exercises performed during strength training.

WHAT YOU WILL NEED:
A wall
If you choose to film yourself to check your form visually afterward, you'll need your phone or a camera

DURATION:
Set aside 15 minutes for your first session and less as you grow more familiar with the movement
Plan to practice this three times a week for two to three weeks

1. Set up your camera to film yourself from the side if you are using one. Do not use a mirror to check your form. Focusing on how the form looks rather than feels runs counter to practicing embodied movement. (Filming provides visual feedback without affecting form, as you'll be watching yourself later on.)

2. Start by standing six inches away from the wall with your back toward it and your feet pointed forward, positioned under your hip joints—not the outside curve of your hips, but under the little bumps of your pelvis.

3. Square your shoulders and stand tall with a neutral spine. Keeping an upright posture and looking straight ahead (chin neither tucked nor lifted), check in and notice what having a relatively straight back feels like. (The spine, even when you "stand up straight," has a natural curve to it.) Hold this sensation in your awareness. Your weight should be in the center of each foot, right below where you'd tie the laces on your sneakers. If you feel that your weight is mostly near your toes, shift your body back a tiny bit. If you feel it in your heels, shift forward. Once your weight is in your midfoot, take a few seconds to really pay attention to how this feels.

4. Next, press the outside edges of your hands (the pinky side) into your horizontal hip crease, right by those bony bumps, which is where your leg bends if you lift your knee straight up. Try to keep

your back's position in mind as you push your bum back by pressing the edges of your hands into your hip crease. Keep your legs straight as you bend. Keep going until your bum grazes the wall. Do not rest on the wall. If you can't reach it, move your setup an inch or two closer to the wall.

5. In this hinged position, with your bum grazing the wall, check in with your body. Start with your back. Is it still long but now pitched forward at an angle? Does it feel the way it felt when you were standing up straight?

6. Next check your feet. Where is your weight? If it shifted backward or forward, find your midfoot again.

7. Now check in with your knees. Are they bent? If so, try to straighten them without locking them.

8. Lastly, check in with your hamstrings, which are the muscles running along the backs of your thighs. Are they taut? They should be, as these muscles are extended when you bend in a hip hinge.

9. At this point you may be fatigued, but before you stand up, let's make sure to come out of the hinge mindfully. Start by contracting your glutes (remember, it feels like trying not to pass gas) and keep squeezing as you push the front of your hips into the edges of your hands, which are still wedged into your hip crease. As you drive up against your hands, keep your attention on your back. Try not to let it round into a c-shape or a bend at the top. Staying with your back and squeezing your bum, slowly come up.

10. Rest and repeat up to three more times.

11. Going forward, stay with this exercise until you're able to graze the wall without losing the weight balance in your feet or bending your back. While you're not lifting any weight, you are still strengthening your muscles and training your nervous system to efficiently bend and lift using your glutes and legs, rather than your back. And the mindfulness alone will mean that you're practicing to lift heavy things.

CHAPTER EIGHT

Claiming Your Agency

E ARLY ON IN MY WORK with private clients, I was stunned by how often they would thank me for listening to them, for centering our sessions on their experiences, preferences, and desire to act on their own behalf. I work this way because empowering the survivor is central to healing from trauma. One private client who earnestly thanked me for listening was Sarah, who you met in Chapter Five. She was by no means meek, nor had she ever seemed hesitant to ask for what she needed from me. I suspect she brought this strength into the rest of her world; she ran her own business and had a rich and fulfilling social life, strong ties to her family and community, and a profoundly deep spiritual practice.

"Thank you for this. I wanted a trainer who believed me, that paying attention to my breath makes me anxious," she said as we wrapped up her session for the day.

Sarah was sitting on the rowing machine in gray sweatpants and a faded dark blue concert t-shirt from years ago. Her hair was pulled into a big bun on top of her head. She had just finished rowing for five minutes while chatting with me, which was one of the ways (rowing or walking on the treadmill, the choice was hers) she'd transition from the activated state of exercise into a calmer state, leaving her more centered in her window of tolerance before she moved on to the next part of her day. Not once did I ask her to pay attention to her breath to find calm, because I already knew she had anxiety around experiencing her breath. She had told me as much when she initially reached out to work with me. She had read an article I'd written, "Why 'Take a Deep Breath' Can Be Terrible Advice," in which I explained why focusing on their breathing can be triggering for some people and provided alternative solutions for calming down.

"You're welcome," I said. I felt a flurry of emotions. I was happy to have been able to help her, but sad that someone would have to feel gratitude for being met with understanding in the gym. This is a right that should be respected, although my own experience has confirmed it isn't always so.

I extended my hands and leveraged my weight to help her up. Standing a head shorter than me, she looked up and smiled with her whole face, including her eyes.

Since then, I've heard this kind of thing many times. Personal training and group coaching clients have said, "Ugh, thank you for not insisting we keep going," "Thank you for caring about me," and my favorite: "You're, like, the nice trainer."

These are all true. I don't push. I do care. And I am nice. What all of these clients were responding to was my regular request that they check in with themselves, be in conversation with their body through their interoceptive experience, and not override their body's signals. What they named "nice" and "caring" is what I do best when I work with folks—create the space for people to be nice and caring to themselves. As for not pushing, I encourage people to listen closely, dig deep, and do hard things only if their body tells them it is okay to.

WHY AGENCY MATTERS

It is vital to your own practice and healing that you cultivate interoception, learn how to be in regular conversation with your body, and take action based on your own experience of it, because that fosters agency. Sarah came to me with a developed sense of interoception and some ideas of what she needed to take better care of herself, and what she needed from me was a trainer who supported her exploration of that. She wanted the tools to allow her to be in conversation with her body and to not override it. As mentioned in Chapter Five, she was working to get back in touch with her body following a trauma, so that she could feel confident enough to train injury-free in group fitness classes. Group fitness can overwhelm you if you aren't ready for the pace or intensity, or if you don't feel empowered to take a break or leave when you have had enough, even if the rest of the class is continuing. With private instruction, I'm able to collaborate with my clients and be curious about their edges, including when and why they express a need to pause or stop. Strength training sustainably for your wellbeing does not demand crushing yourself. Pain is a signal that should be honored, not overridden, just like fears and insecurities around being in the gym should be addressed, not ignored. Yet what I see in many mainstream fitness classes and professionals is the opposite: an unyielding, aggressive pushing through pain and fear of any kind. These trainers view reasons for stopping as excuses or weaknesses, and deem them off-limits.

With Sarah, I could see the high school athlete she had once been right away in her approach to movement, and I was pleased she had this inner resource for a number of reasons. I often play catch with my clients using a large, weighted ball called a medicine ball. Clients who, like me, fell through the cracks of PE, often need to be taught how to throw efficiently by putting their whole body behind a chest pass. However, when I passed Sarah the ball, her inner athlete caught it with a playful glint in her eye and a solid pass of the four-pound ball back to me. High school may have been nearly half her lifetime ago, but she was still an athlete—and maybe even more athletic than her trainer.

At the same time, she could feel constriction inside her body when she went to inhale deeply (paying attention through interoception). When she reported it to previous fitness professionals, they would disregard it, either by minimizing it as "nothing" or by encouraging her to just push through. She wanted the opportunity to honor and address the constriction and I was able to give her that.

Your agency is your capacity to act independently and to make your own free choices. Part of the capacity to act is being able to know what you want and need. Interoception, or being able to feel what's happening inside ourselves, is crucial to this knowing. If I ignored my clients' experience of their bodies, insisting that deep breathing will work, that they push through pain, or move in ways they object to, I would be undermining one of the major tenets of my practice: to help people identify what they want and need, and when, and to feel empowered to take the action necessary to get there. My client, an expert in herself, came to me with this knowing, which isn't something everyone has (not necessarily even the most embodied of folks). It was my job to get her to train while staying curious about it.

So instead of pushing and ignoring what she knew to be true of her experience, she and I worked together on getting stronger slowly and steadily. We honored her interoceptive experience while alternating between her strengths (chest passes, squats, and deadlifts) and movements that were harder and created more arousal (like hamstring curls and lat pull downs). She progressed each week, slowly increasing the amount of weight she lifted or reps she completed. We went slowly so that she'd feel comfortable and able to get back into her window of tolerance easily should she feel triggered, whether by the movement in a dissociated body part or any other arousal from exercise, including breathing. I tracked all that information as we went and would show her when she asked to review it, as I do with all my clients.

HOW AGENCY AIDS IN HEALING

Experiencing your agency is potent and can set the stage for personal change and growth. It is also fundamental to healing trauma. Dr. Judith Herman notes that "the empowerment of the survivor" is central to recovery from trauma, that "[they] must be the author and arbiter of [their] own recovery."[1]

As such, I don't only structure workouts to help people connect with their body so they can identify what it's asking of them through interoception; I give them the opportunity to pursue those wants or needs using two-way communication, which in the specific case of my work means always using invitational language, asking for and obtaining consent throughout each workout, and engaging in active listening. And while I'm not working one-on-one with you right now in a physical sense, I want to share my knowledge of these things with you so you can look for them in any practitioner you include on your healing path, and ask for them from whomever you choose to work with going forward. While I know plenty of fitness professionals who don't do these things, I also know quite a few who do.

You are an expert in yourself. You, and only you, have had your unique lived experience. Using interoception to determine what you want and need is only half the equation—you then need to take that knowledge and act on your own behalf, guided by what will truly serve you best. People who deny your experience and ignore your boundaries (more of which in the next chapter) are manipulating you into questioning your truth. They may be doing so with the intention of helping you, but in denying you your true feelings, thoughts, and experiences, they are undermining any "greater good" they seek to provide. As a helper, my role is clear: to assist you with my expertise in listening to the body and the different paths to healing.

With a client, I actively listen and strive to deeply understand their experience while we simultaneously hold it as theirs alone, separate from my own. I make space to honor their lived experience because everyone deserves to be seen and heard, though not everyone is. The strategies I've included below are a few ways you can start to recognize active listening in your own communication as well as others', as indications of honoring mutual agency on all sides.

Invitational Language

Invitational language presents the opportunity for the client to engage with something—trying a new movement, taking a break, or even starting training. I always ask my clients, "Are you ready to strength train today?" as opposed to telling them, "It's time to train." I say to them, "I have you programmed for squats today, does that feel okay for you?" instead of telling them, "Today is a squat day." And then I listen for their answer.

Most of the time my clients say yes, but sometimes they say no, and both are great answers. While it means tweaking the program I planned, "no" is an opportunity for us to have a conversation in which I respect my client's wishes and get curious with them about their response, possible fears, or reservations. I ask them why they don't want to do the exercise and then we have a discussion about it. Maybe it's hurting their body in some way. If so, I might suggest an adjustment, to which they may say yes or no, and then we take it from there. It's not a debate. There is nothing to "win." My clients are not just doing the work of getting fit; they're doing the work of healing, learning interoception, setting boundaries, and finding agency. This all allows them to be seen and heard in their wholeness.

Asking For and Obtaining Consent

Along the same lines as using invitational language, I ask for consent each time I go to touch a client and I wait for a positive verbal and physical response before doing so. And like using invitational language, this too can feel cumbersome at first. But the fact is that people are sometimes okay with being touched and other times they are not. A client may feel differently on different days, or even within the course of a session. When I encounter a client who says something along the lines of, "It's always okay, you don't have to ask each time," I say, "I am going to ask you each time, just in case." I want to stress that no matter the practitioner and modality you're working with, you always have the right to say yes or no to touch, even if you are not asked.

Active Listening

In all of these examples, I have talked not only about asking questions of my clients, but really listening to their answers. Wellness practitioners, myself included, are often eager to help people by offering advice; the downside of this is, in our eagerness, we risk forgetting to take the time to gather all the information needed to offer the best possible advice. If a client says "I don't want to squat because it hurts my knee," I may be inclined to try to quickly solve the problem based on my own experience with squats and knee pain. But if I do that, I'm working with my experience, not theirs, and what works for me or another client may not work for them. Furthermore, "It hurts my knee" is a little vague, and I'd need more information about their personal experience with knee pain. What's the quality and location of the pain, and when is it triggered? What, if anything, makes it better? Is this pain an old companion, or a new and scary one? While I'm not diagnosing the cause of the pain, I am assessing it and determining if there can be a way to train a particular muscle, or group of muscles, in such a way as to not cause more aggravation and maybe even help to alleviate it.

Two-way communication does a number of things, but at its core, it gives folks the opportunity to practice using interoception and to take action on their own behalf using the information garnered from their interoceptive experience.

Counselors and therapists across different schools of psychotherapy agree that agency—feeling able to act on behalf of oneself—is essential to sound mental health. Although I'm not a licensed mental health practitioner, I believe that as a trauma-informed personal trainer seeking to foster conditions that heal mind, body, and spirit, I must give my clients every opportunity to experience acting out of their own agency while working with me. This might look like asking for support in pursuing an action ("I want to squat but it hurts my knees. Can we find a way that doesn't hurt?"), or telling me, "I need to stop now." Practicing this while in the gym gives you a solid foundation of experience that you can take with you outside of it, into your home, workplace, and beyond.

If you're using exercise to heal from trauma then you are likely pursuing physical goals, but probably also healing goals, which may include practicing basic self-care. You can't address your needs if you don't know what they are, and you can't know your own needs if you cannot feel them. And when you're overwhelmed by stress and have been thrust outside your window of tolerance, you will likely flee your body in one way or another and not have access to that embodied knowing. Like the athlete who overrides injury under the stress of performance, it's easy for people living with trauma to miss the signals the body gives by checking out of it.

I have some clients who often forget to drink water and realize that they're thirsty only when I ask them; other clients don't realize they're free to use the restroom during our session.

Think about the ways in which you neglect your own needs when you're trying to get a project done by a big deadline, working a double shift, or balancing school, work, and family during crunch time. You might push yourself to stand until your feet and ankles swell, or else sit until your back locks up. You might also skip meals, sleep, and moments of human connection. When I'm working hard and feeling stressed out, I neglect my body's cues for very basic care. I don't realize I have to go to the bathroom until I experience abdominal cramping; I forget to eat until my stomach hurts; I don't realize I am exhausted until my eyes close and I can't see what I'm doing anymore. When all is said and done, we feel rotten when we miss these basic cues from our body to take action.

By staying in touch with your body while you exercise, you will be able to hear it when it tells you what it needs. It's only from this embodied place that you can truly consent to things, like the exercises in the program or an instructor's hands-on correction. If you sense that you need to rest more than is offered, I believe you should rest. If a movement hurts, this is a signal that either the movement, or the way you're performing it, is wrong for you at that time and should be changed. If you show up to the gym but then decide you don't want to train, it's worth exploring potential reasons before you head home, but at the end of the day, it's your call. Most people aren't training to engage in a sport competitively. Even when I train in something sport-centered, like Olympic weightlifting or powerlifting, I no longer sign up for meets. Training for meets doesn't feed any part of me anymore. It once served that purpose, but when I listen to my body now, the message is loud and clear: "I train to manage pain, not override it. I train to feel grounded, not to fight. I train to feel good, not to win."

You, dear reader, are likely also looking for ways to feel good—whatever that means to you—and to support your mental and physical health. Learning to honor your body's signals and stand up for them, not override them in the name of short-term performance, will serve your health and well-being in the long term.

TAKE ACTION
Give Parts of Your Body a Voice

Our bodies talk to us through sensations. So far, we have explored ways to foster the ability to notice these sensations and act accordingly. Sometimes, a particular body part frequently has something to say; maybe it's your knee or shoulder that locks up often, a muscle that frequently spasms, or even a nervous tick. In this exercise, you're going to get to know that part of yourself better by giving it a voice.

WHAT YOU WILL NEED:
A journal or a piece of paper
A writing instrument
A safe-feeling space to write in
A talkative part of your body (one that frequently hurts, cramps, spasms, locks up, twitches or otherwise calls for your attention)

DURATION:
15 minutes or more, after engaging in a session of embodied movement

1. Pick a place to do this exercise that feels safe and supportive. If your movement practice happens in a gym or other public place, you might find a quiet spot to sit in or head out to your car. If you want to wait until you're home, take a few minutes beforehand to mindfully stretch, walk, or do the movements in the Take Action section from Chapter Five, so as to be in an embodied place.

2. Once seated, you're going to do the opposite of the Sounds Near to Far exercise presented at the end of Chapter Four: With your eyes either closed or softly lowered, listen to sounds coming from far away, perhaps from outdoors. Next, listen to sounds closer to you: inside the building you're in, then inside the room. Now listen to the sounds coming from inside you, like breathing and swallowing.

3. When you're ready to hear, ask the concerned body part—either out loud or in your head—"What would you like to tell me?" Write down whatever comes up. You might continue to engage in dialogue with this part of you, or it may be more of a monologue from that part. Spend five to ten minutes writing whatever comes up.

4. At the end of the conversation, thank the body part for what it has shared. When you're ready, intentionally reorient yourself to the room through sound, this time using the original exercise as set out in Chapter Four.

5. Repeat this practice whenever you feel curious about what a part of your body needs and wants to communicate with it so you can take informed action on your own behalf.

CHAPTER NINE
Finding and Restoring Your Boundaries

C LIENTS OFTEN ASSUME, understandably, that fitness and wellness practitioners have been trained in understanding and respecting boundaries with clients, or even that this is an unspoken agreement and such training is not needed. But clients and practitioners both carry their own experiences and relationships to boundaries, and in my opinion, they need to be explicitly addressed. What's more, a student or trainee practitioner may be shaky on the meaning of boundaries.

All this is important to keep in mind when working with trauma, where there has been an inherent breach of boundaries that needs repair. Although many wellness professionals encourage, if not outright instruct you to have boundaries and to enforce them as part of your self-care, I feel compelled to address that this is easier said than done when grappling with trauma.

At the time I began training after [   ], I was struggling with boundaries on all sides. I grew up in environments where boundaries weren't properly modelled, so I didn't know what they were until I started my healing work, well into my thirties. I also experienced emotional and physical trauma over the years, which damaged whatever boundaries I did have. By the time [   ] occurred, I felt very porous, which made it hard for me to understand where I ended and others began. Not knowing my edges made me feel unsafe even when socializing with friends whom I knew, trusted, and liked.

One Wednesday afternoon at the end of March, I arrived early to meet my friend Rachel at a lunch spot in the city—a nondescript sort of place which I remember as very beige, white, and boring. The restaurant was long and narrow, and the host let me wait at our table right in the center of the space. With my back to the wall, I was able to survey the room. For about ten minutes, I would lean forward, look left to the door, turn my head, look right to the back, and sit back. I would look down at my phone, which was unconsciously clutched in my hands, tap around on it mindlessly for a bit, and look up again.

It had been two months since [   ] and less than one month since I'd told someone what happened. I was still trying to act as if I were okay. It was an act that came to a close only when my back went out seven months later and I struggled to get out of bed. The fact was, I didn't trust that anyone would meet me with support and care in this situation, and I was too vulnerable to reach out with anything less than unconditional trust. Advice felt too overwhelming and criticism impossible to bear. I just wanted to be seen and heard, but people—often the well-meaning ones—try to do more than listen: they try to fix things even when they can't. Right then, it felt like if someone did anything more than just hold space for me, including trying to fix things, I might break. That would be fairly easy, as I walked around feeling brittle constantly. If I was pushed slightly, I felt as if I would shatter, letting my contents come spilling out and overwhelming everyone around me. I would be too much. They would leave me. This was my boundary: brittle and fragile, but so important to my survival.

In hindsight, I know that I am not "too much," and wasn't then, either. But it took years for me to embody this thought at all, and in fact, it's still not anchored to my foundation so securely.

I had never met Rachel for lunch in the city before. We knew each other from summer trips to a small island about two hours' drive from the city, comprising a handful of towns that attract queer people, Jewish families, and middle and upper-class families. My family has been going there to visit for three generations. It's beautiful and I loved it as a teenager. But as an adult, I've never really had a great time there. Rachel couldn't fathom this because it's one of her favorite places on earth.

I like Rachel a lot. She's very fun, fiery, funny, tough, and has an opinion on everything. Although the timing wasn't great for a chatty lunch with a new friend, I was grasping for a sense of normalcy, which to me included lunch dates. However, I knew that in my moment of crisis, I wouldn't be able to handle her opinion on what happened to me or how I was responding to it. In the spirit of keeping things light, I decided the night before that I wouldn't tell her about [   ], and reaffirmed that decision to myself as I watched her walk in and say something to the host that made them both laugh.

I got up as she walked over. We hugged and sat down at our table, and we began to catch up as if everything was normal.

"Are you going to come out to the beach this summer?" Rachel asked.

"I don't think so," I replied.

"Why? You should come. It's so nice. You'll love it," she carried on. But I knew that I would not love it. After [   ], I was too scared to travel and be away from my cats and my bed, to go to a place I never really felt comfortable in even though my friends out there insisted I should "love it."

"I don't know. I have some things going on and I just don't think I'll be up to it," I said, trying to push away her opinions.

"What's going on?" she asked, her face softening and eyes opening up as if to take all of me in. Her tone, more gentle now, conveyed some worry. She was genuinely concerned.

"Something happened. I don't want to talk about it," I said, my insides pushing against my edges. I clutched my napkin with both fists in my lap and pressed the balls of my feet into the ground, bracing myself. I did not want to tell the story. I didn't like telling people. I had told those who needed to know and a few others from whom I sought support, like my husband, therapist, and a few close friends.

"Oh c'mon. Tell me. You can tell me," she began to pry, needling at my brittle boundary. Inside, I tried to make my contents smaller by squeezing tighter, but I couldn't stop feeling myself pressing against my outsides. This was my boundary. I was aware of it, as thin and fragile as it was, and I knew it was under attack.

"No," I said quietly, shaking my head and looking down.

Then she began to guess and kept guessing until she hit the nail on the head, shattering my boundary into a million pieces just as I'd feared. She then tried to tell me what I should do by telling me what she would do, and that what I had done so far was wrong. This torrent of advice was coming from her experience of her own life, not from an experience of mine. This was sympathy without empathy. She was trying to be a good friend and she wasn't succeeding.

I left that lunch shattered and shaken, feeling so vulnerable and anything but normal—the opposite of what I needed to make myself whole again.

I invite you to pause and check in with your-
self, and assess if you need anything right now. If
you do, please tend to yourself accordingly.

WHY BOUNDARIES MATTER

With trauma, no matter your individual story, comes a breach of your boundaries. Boundaries are where you end and the rest of the energetic, emotional, and physical world begins. They are the edges that contain you. Your skin contains your skeleton and viscera, your energy field contains your energetic being, and your emotional field contains your emotions. Maybe that breach occurred slowly, like rust eating away a hole, or more quickly, like a tire puncture. In physical trauma, the breach is more obvious. It might be a wound sustained in a fall that breaks your visible boundary, your skin. The same could be said for diseases, which are often spoken about like invaders of the body. Accidents and surgeries, even elective ones, involve a breach of our physical boundary as well.

In emotional trauma, the breach isn't visible to the eye, but it very much exists. Emotional boundaries separate you and your feelings from another person's. Divorce, neglect, verbal abuse, and bullying can all lead to emotional trauma. Non-physical violations spurred on by racism, homophobia, misogyny, xenophobia, ableism, and ageism are also emotionally traumatic. In these cases, even if no one puts their hands on you, their behavior is injurious. Some traumas, such as experiencing assault or rape, involve breaches to both our physical and emotional boundaries.

Having a sense of your boundaries following a trauma and feeling equipped to enforce them allows you to move about the world feeling safer, and this comes from moments of being embodied. You'll know where your edges are, what belongs to you, and what belongs outside of you. Other people's judgments will be less easily internalized, even if it's still uncomfortable. When people and events push up against your edges, you'll be better able to feel them, including if those edges are about to give. This level of certainty about your boundaries can only come from really feeling them through practice. Certainty can fuel brave actions, like saying "no" or "things have to change" or "I'm leaving," even if you've spent prior months or maybe even years sucking it up and numbing the pain. This could also look like standing up to a parent who still tells you how to live your life as an adult, a friend or co-worker who takes advantage of you, or a partner who disrespects you. It's never too late to discover your boundaries, or demand that others respect them.

Being perceptive of your boundaries also means that you'll be able to tell when you are running on empty. You may catch yourself saying things like, "I'm drained," "I don't have anything left in the tank," or "I'm exhausted." You may notice that you feel like you're dragging yourself to your next task, as if you have weight on your shoulders. When this happens, it's time to honor your boundaries by replenishing them and to tend to yourself by doing something you find restorative. Caregivers, activists, and people in the helping professions are all familiar with this feeling.

All sorts of things can be restorative: engaging in a spiritual practice, getting pampered, seeking counseling, playing a game with people you love, eating or cooking a meal you enjoy, practicing gentle yoga, curling up with a good book, baking, meeting up with a friend, or going for a walk are the ideal self-care activities that come to mind for myself. As with embodied movement, what you do is not as important as the way you do it. This restoration may have an element of mindfulness to it, but it doesn't have to. The activity should nourish your spirit or body (or both!). The intention behind engaging in self-care or community care (in which people come together to care for one another as a group) is to leave feeling rested, like you have the energy to tackle whatever comes next. Life happens. We can't avoid stressors altogether, but we can manage our energy levels to some extent.

EMBODIMENT AND BOUNDARIES

Although the work we've already done together in this book will lay the foundations, finding and honoring your boundaries takes practice. It's a way to enforce your sense of agency, which in turn makes you feel you have the right and means to protect your boundaries. We all face challenges to our boundaries regularly. Maybe your boss asks you to come in on your day off yet again, or your parents undermine your own parenting by ignoring the rules you set for your children. Or maybe you have a friend or partner who, like Rachel, can pry and be pushy, not because they have bad intentions but because they care. Are you able to advocate for yourself when these things happen? Perhaps, but for lots of folks who've had their boundaries violated, or else never learned to recognize them, this can be very hard.

I had been actively trying to heal from trauma for over two years before I stood up for myself and my values in the gym. Tired of lifting heavy things in an atmosphere where objectifying women was okay and it was assumed everyone was primarily pursuing leanness, I requested a decrease in conversation about clients' and athletes' appearance. When my requests were dismissed, I cut ties with the gym and coaches alike, letting them know why in no uncertain terms.

Before that moment, I'd been practicing self-awareness enough to be able to notice my boundaries. I challenged myself to ask for help. I sought the care I needed to heal the broken barrier of my container and fill it up with energy. This was all hard work, but it didn't last forever and the payoff was huge. Leaving that gym was a major step toward finding my power and my own voice in the fitness community.

TAKE ACTION
Push Away

All strength exercises involve a push, a pull, or sometimes both, and training in both actions is important for your physical health and wellbeing. Pushing can teach us how to say no with our bodies, while pulling can teach us how to reach out and ask for more, which is just another form of agency.

My clients often have a hard time feeling into their boundaries and are uncertain of what it feels like to push away requests and demands that impinge on them. For those clients, we work on literal pushing as a way to practice that kind of interoception and action impulse across other areas of their lives.

WHAT YOU WILL NEED:
A wall
A journal or a piece of paper
A writing instrument

DURATION:
5 minutes

1. Stand facing a wall at arm's length. Reach forward and place your palms on the wall, slightly wider than shoulder-width apart.

2. Bend your elbows, bringing your body close to the wall like in a half push-up. Your elbows should bend so that your upper arms make a 45-degree angle (or smaller) with your body. Support yourself by lightly contracting your glutes and abs.

3. I invite you to notice how close the wall is and feel it meeting the palms of your hands. Notice which sensations come up in your body.

4. When you're ready, shove the wall away from you with just enough force to stand up. If you push so hard you fall backward a bit, practice controlling your push to find the right amount of effort to come to a stable standing position.

5. Once upright, I invite you to take a moment to notice the space between you and the wall again. Notice any shifts in your body.

6. Repeat three to five times.

7. Take a few minutes to record your experience and any meaning or observations you make of it. If you are in therapy, it may be helpful to process the experience of doing this exercise with your therapist.

PART III
RECOVERY

Resilience, which is built during recovery,
is the ability to return to rest with ease
after lifting heavy things—not simply
the ability to tolerate lifting them.

CHAPTER TEN

Increasing Your Resilience with Recovery

THE FIRST TIME I EVER ENCOUNTERED a "cool down" was in the mid-'80s, at my grandmother's sprawling, pre-war apartment on the Upper East Side of Manhattan. A cool down is the final, least intense section of a high-intensity workout, which transitions your body from working hard to recovery. While some people are tempted to skip the cool down, I advise sticking around for it as it serves a number of purposes: it prevents blood from pooling and causing dizziness, which can happen when you suddenly go from high levels of exertion to none at all; it reduces post-workout muscle soreness; and it eases you back into your resting state, closer to the middle of your window of tolerance.

But six-year-old me didn't know any of that. I just knew that after the cool down, I felt good.

I was very close with my maternal grandmother, Gloria, who passed away in 2006, leaving a giant hole in the fabric of my little family. When I was growing up, she would visit me in the suburbs every week, even buying a car and learning to drive it for that very purpose. And I would regularly visit her in the city. She'd take me to see new exhibitions at the Museum of Modern Art, to tea at The Pierre or The Plaza Hotel, and toy shopping at FAO Schwarz (I almost never wanted anything from there and would also request a trip to my favorite store, Woolworth's, a five-and-dime with toys that left more to the imagination, which I preferred). We would have lunch at Burger Heaven, like the characters in Judy Blume's *Tales of a Fourth Grade Nothing*, or at the Automat, after I learned about it but before the last one closed. I was fascinated by selecting food from behind little windows. Then we would go to the playground in Central Park and have dinner at John's Pizza or JG Melon. I loved my visits with my grandmother.

Her living room was large enough for two seating areas, a writing desk, and a piano, but it had no TV as she did not believe in keeping one in the living room. But she did have TVs—four, in fact. Small black-and-white models could be found in the kitchen and den. Another television was in my uncle John's bedroom. He was autistic, lived with Gloria for most of his adult life, and would watch a lot of TV when he returned home from his various restaurant jobs.

The fourth TV, a larger color model, was kept in her unusually large foyer, which doubled as a TV room. Like much of the apartment, this room's mid-century modern furniture juxtaposed pleasantly with its pre-war architectural bones. There were two small settees placed kitty-corner to one another at one end of the room, and a wooden accent table with a decorative lip on its rounded corners nestled between them. Two small wood and brass tables stood on the black and white rug that covered the black-speckled tile floor beneath. Across from the sitting area were two credenzas in which my grandmother kept her collection of silk scarves and cashmere hats and gloves. The remotes for the television and VCR were kept in a drawer, and the television and VCR were kept on a separate rollaway cart, unobtrusively tucked in across from the settees. When I wasn't busy acting out fantasies of saving myself from my library-ladder-cum-castle tower in the living room, or of saving my stuffed animal from a shipwreck in the den, I was in the foyer watching TV.

Among my grandmother's few VHS tapes, most of which I remember being blank tapes on which she'd recorded PBS programs, was *Jane Fonda's Workout*. I had no idea who Jane Fonda was, but I immediately fell in love with everything she was about. I was wooed by her soft curls and her smile, her fuchsia and purple candy-cane striped leotard with coordinating belt, tights, and leg warmers. Fascinated by the lady on the box, I asked my grandmother about the tape and she encouraged me to try it. At six years old, I had yet to feel self-conscious of my body or be made fun of in gym class. In fact, I loved being in my body. I would dance and play unencumbered by judgment. And so, without reservation, I did *Jane Fonda's Workout* and really enjoyed myself. I don't ever remember seeing my grandmother in workout clothes doing it when I visited, but she must have followed along herself at some point. For the next few years, until my "everything-adults-do-is-lame" mentality set in, I would do *Jane Fonda's Workout* whenever I visited my grandmother for a sleepover, and the energy behind it has stayed with me until today.

I was hooked from the very beginning, when Jane (I just thought of her as my teacher Jane, first-name basis) first asked the group of women and men dressed in color-blocked leotards, tights, and legwarmers, "Are you ready to do the workout?" then turned to the camera and asked me "Are *you* ready to do the workout?" We stomped, clapped, and snapped to the synthesized music. We circled our arms, ran in place, raised our legs, and squeezed our bums in time to the rhythm. We pulsed and circled and swung our bodies at every joint, moving all around the room. And we celebrated working out, like we were at one big party. The people in the background would let out impromptu hoots and exclaim, "Yeah!" and Jane would remind us to "Feel that burn!" Scissoring my arms up and down was my favorite move. I got to wiggle my hips and swing my arms up and down and side to side. Even as a kid, the ab work toward the end was my least favorite part, but I did it because I wanted to be like the grown-ups in the video with their fluffy hair, amazing spandex outfits, and graceful movements.

As much as I liked the energy of doing aerobics, my very favorite part was at the end of the workout, when Jane instructed the class to come into a shoulder stand—an inversion where you lie on your back and stretch your legs straight up to the ceiling, toes pointed, with your bum and back off the floor so your weight is on your shoulders. This was the cue for her to say, "This is the cool down portion of the program." After nearly thirty minutes of "feeling that burn," I was thrilled to come into a shoulder stand and then, in bendy little kid fashion, easily extend my straightened legs back until my toes touched the ground behind my head.

From this position, Jane instructed me to relax my spine, shoulder blades, and forehead, and to breathe. She dropped her knees beside her ears and breathed, and so did I. Then she would straighten her knees and hold her ankles, and we would slowly lower our legs together, "one vertebra at a time," until we were lying on our backs with our knees tucked into our chests.

"Shh," Jane said, before prompting me to sit up slowly. We would then come up to stand on our feet and stay folded over "like a rag doll." Finally, we would slowly unroll again, one vertebra at a time. The camera moved above her so she was looking up at me, her full curls framing her smiling face, glowing with the rush of exercise-induced endorphins as she guided me through head rolls and deep breaths. And then she'd say to me, "You did a great job. Don't you feel good?"

"Yes," I would answer, out loud and with pride. While I knew she couldn't see me or hear me, I felt seen and heard. I did do a great job, and I did feel good! As an only child and only grandchild, I gladly accepted pre-recorded validation as I was often alone. Jane had gotten my heart rate up, my endorphins pumping, and made my muscles burn, which resulted in an aliveness that I seldom got in the TV room watching cartoons and gameshows. Then she would ease me back into my day again, so I could keep playing 'the floor is water' and all sorts of other imaginative games.

COOL DOWN FOR HEAVY LIFTING

Rest and recovery, which Jane Fonda offered as part of her cool down, are important parts of both practicing and healing. In addition to increasing your capacity for stress, healing work can also mean practicing recovering from stress with greater ease. You do this through intentionally engaging in rest after intentionally engaging in arousal.

Your nervous system is aroused while you're doing the work of activation, and you use that arousal to drive physical development. You're building neural connections and preparing your body to strengthen its muscles and bones. You may feel more hungry or tired at bedtime on the days you engage in your movement practice. This is your body saying, "Hey, I need resources to replenish, grow, and change." You gather those resources during rest and recovery.

It's not until you rest that your body takes all the lessons it's learned in the gym, on your bike, or at the rock wall, and integrates those developments. Your muscles don't get stronger the moment you lift heavy things—they get stronger as they recover *after* you lift them. And your body doesn't get more efficient during the time you spend training, but afterwards, based on what you did in your training and how.

The same can be said about processing trauma. While you are processing it, in the therapist's office, on a hike, or while journaling, you are aroused and will likely feel some of the same sensations you experienced during your trauma. Afterward, you'll need to rest and take time to integrate any changes in perspective or new understandings you may have.

After I engage in a strength workout now, I often use a combination of forward folds and active recovery to reset my nervous system. Forward folds stimulate the parasympathetic nervous system, also known as the "rest and digest" system. This signals to your body that it's time to move away from the stress response induced by exercise (Jane Fonda knew what she was doing). Those five or ten minutes that some people like to skip (myself included on some days) actively encourage a rest response, so that you're ready to recover and to increase your strength and nervous system's resilience. When something is resilient, it's able to return to the baseline with ease.

COOL DOWN FOR RESILIENCE

Stress is unavoidable. Conflicts with loved ones or colleagues, navigating life changes like moving and divorce, and receiving heartbreaking news, are all common events that increase nervous system arousal. This in turn releases stress hormones, creating tension in the muscles, increasing our heart rate, and heightening sensitivity in all areas. These stress responses consume a lot of energy so you're likely to feel depleted afterward, just like after lifting heavy things at the gym.

A resilient nervous system is not one that doesn't experience stress at all, but one that can recover from stress and the accompanying energy expenditure more quickly, with a natural rhythm. If your nervous system is less resilient, it will be harder to move between arousal and rest. But remember: you can practice. And to do so, you must practice coming in and out of both states.

Jane Fonda understood the importance of both arousal and rest. Her workout tape offers a beginner program and an advanced program, and the user is encouraged to go at their own pace. Both start by slowly increasing your arousal with a warm-up, followed by targeted work on the arms, trunk, and legs, and then the cool down. By going at your own pace, you honor how much activation you want to engage in so that you don't overextend yourself. Jane guides your activation to the edge of your window of tolerance and gives you tools to come back down toward the end.

Being comfortable with rest takes time and may even feel unattainable or scary. While many of my clients like to lie down and do guided stretches at the end of a workout, or even receive some energy work, I've had other clients who found that absolutely intolerable. I know I've had periods when I felt this way as well, keeping myself busy with tasks despite being exhausted because traditional forms of rest ask for stillness. Intentional stillness can prompt a feeling of vulnerability too big to tolerate. It can remind you of times when you felt immobilized under threat. It can even trigger anxiety and panic attacks.

Beyond these experiences on a personal level, American culture itself praises action over rest. People will always applaud your ability to do more but rarely will you receive congratulations for managing to get adequate rest (I've probably never received as much praise from my friends and community as when I was training ten times a week). When it comes to our nervous system's automatic responses to threat, many people think "fight" or "flight" is somehow more noble than "freeze." We feel shame if we didn't get away or fight off the bad guy. In truth, we have all evolved to do whatever saves our lives, and that is awesome.

The good news is that there is a lot of room between staying busy, training relentlessly, and stillness, just like there's a continuum of arousal from complete rest to intense activity that can be explored in a cool down.

A key to finding rest when you find it difficult to stop moving is to engage in moderate activity, sometimes referred to as active recovery. Walking, hiking, and certain forms of yoga are all ways to move your body while also encouraging your nervous system to move into a rest state. You can encourage rest with any movement practice that takes work but still allows you to breathe through your nose and talk. Think back to my client Sarah, who liked to end her sessions rowing or on the treadmill. She was moving and recovering at the same time. If stillness is hard, this approach will help you feel better in the present and allow you to handle the ordinary stresses of life, bigger stresses, and even trauma more easily in the future.

Steady-state cardio is exercise that gets your heart rate up, which you then keep up for the duration of the session, as opposed to something like interval training, which pendulates your heart rate by bringing it up and then back down. For recovery purposes, the heart rate sustained should be a moderate one, which I'll tell you how to calculate in the Take Action portion of this chapter. If you don't have a heart rate monitor, you can achieve a moderate heart rate by working just hard enough that it feels like work—you may just break a sweat, your breathing becomes more pronounced—but not so hard that you can't carry on a conversation. If seasonal allergies or a cold make breathing through your nose difficult, that's okay, but you should not be panting.

And again, just to clarify, rest is different from collapsing from exhaustion. Collapse means you have depleted yourself and your body is going into emergency reserves. When you are at rest, your body is still at work integrating all the things you're learning, processing, and developing. Collapse allows for survival, while rest allows for recovery. Surviving is good, but only recovery makes space for thriving.

Jane Fonda didn't just leave me alone to rest after all that aerobic stimulation—she guided me from arousal into rest through a series of quieting movements that made me feel my vitality. She set me up to recover. Now I'd like to do the same for you.

TAKE ACTION
Steady-State Cardio for Active Recovery

Getting your body ready to recover after the stress of a workout, or even the stress of a hard day, is an important practice for promoting a healthy nervous system. Steady-state cardio is an excellent active way to do this, and I often use it as a form of active recovery with my clients.

If you're doing this as a cool down at the end of your workout, ten minutes is a great duration to start with. Of course, if ten minutes feels like too much work, start with less and work toward ten minutes. Add an additional minute each week, or every two to three sessions, until you get to ten.

You can also use steady-state cardio as a standalone practice. I often encourage clients with high-stress lives, chronic fatigue syndrome, or sleep disorders, to go for walks, do some yoga, or take a twenty-minute bike ride on days they don't strength train. This practice encourages the nervous system to move from a slightly aroused state to a restful one. For caregivers or people who want to use their free time to socialize, I suggest you bring along someone who is interested in joining you, which can further add to the restorative nature of the activity.

Not everyone can find relaxation in stillness. If this is you, or you're having trouble finding relaxation and haven't given cardio exercise a try,

I suggest you try this out for a couple of weeks and see how you feel after a workout and on non-training days.

In this exercise, I provide two options for determining how hard to work while engaging in steady-state cardio. In Option A, you'll calculate your target heart rate with a heart rate monitor or other piece of cardio equipment that measures heart rate. In Option B, you'll use breath as a way to monitor effort. I'm providing both options because some people find it regulating to have set metrics to use, while others find calculations and equipment overwhelming. Choose the option that works best for you. Once you have your target steady-state heart rate range, you should engage in an activity that allows you to stay in this range for the duration.

OPTION A: CALCULATE YOUR TARGET HEART RATE RANGE USING A HEART MONITOR

WHAT YOU WILL NEED:
A calculator, or paper and writing instrument to do calculations
A cardio modality (advice to help you pick one is below)
A heart rate monitor

DURATION:
10 or more minutes
An additional 5 minutes the first time you do this to calculate your target heart rate

Start by finding your resting heart rate (HRrest). The best way to do this is to take your pulse first thing when you wake up, while you are still lying in bed. Place the pads of your pointer finger and middle finger of your left hand on your pulse point on your right wrist or right side of your neck. Count your heartbeats for 10 seconds. Multiply that by 6. That is your resting heart rate.

Pulse count after you wake for 10 seconds × 6 = HRrest

Write your HRrest down somewhere you can refer to it later.

Next, find your maximum heart rate (HRmax) by subtracting your age from 220.

$$220 - your\ age = HRmax$$

Next subtract your HRrest from your HRmax to calculate what is known as your heart rate reserve (HRR), a number which represents the range of your heart rate.

$$HRmax - HRrest = HRR$$

To calculate a heart rate target for steady-state cardio, you would take 40 percent of your HRR and add it to your HRrest. Then take half of your HRR and add it to your HRrest. These two numbers represent the bottom and top of your range for steady-state cardio.

$$(0.4 \times HRR) + HRrest = bottom\ of\ target\ range$$

$$(0.5 \times HRR) + HRrest = top\ of\ target\ range$$

For example, a forty-five-year-old who wakes up with a heart rate of 65 beats per minute (bpm) would calculate their steady state cardio range like this:

$$220 - 45 = HRmax\ of\ 175$$

$$175 - 65 = HRR\ of\ 110$$

$$(0.4 \times 110) + 65 = Bottom\ of\ target\ range\ is\ 109$$

$$(0.5 \times 110) + 65 = Top\ of\ target\ range\ is\ 120$$

Their steady state target range is: 109–120 bpm

OPTION B: USE BREATH TO MONITOR WORK LEVELS

WHAT YOU WILL NEED:
A cardio modality (advice to help you pick one is below)

DURATION:
10 or more minutes

As a guide to choosing an activity appropriate for recovery purposes, you'll want to get your body working, but not breathing too hard to carry on a conversation. Now that you're working at a pace that allows for this, engage in an activity that allows you to stay in this range for the duration.

SUGGESTIONS FOR USING STEADY-STATE ACTIVITY FOR BOTH OPTIONS A AND B

If you do this as a cool down after a workout, plan to spend ten minutes doing steady-state cardio. You could use cardio training equipment of any kind, or walk a track around a park, the neighborhood, or a shopping mall. You could walk part or all of your commute, or bike it; you could swim, or walk the stairs in your apartment or office building. Pick something you can do at a steady pace for at least ten minutes, working hard yet still able to talk. If you can breathe through your nose easily then I encourage you to do so, as this will help calm your nervous system. And if you find yourself breathing too hard to talk, then pick something less challenging.

For a standalone workout, start with ten minutes and aim to increase this by five minutes each week until you've reached thirty minutes or more.

CHAPTER ELEVEN
Start Somewhere

MANY OF MY FRIENDS AND FAMILY MEMBERS who aren't into fitness have asked me, "How do you do it?" Even my chatty ophthalmologist, Dr. Friedman, asks me about the gym. He is very friendly, loves his work, and—as I have learned—hates going to the gym himself. Our conversation during my appointment in August 2017 followed familiar lines.

"You're still bodybuilding?" Dr. Friedman inquired as he held my eye open and peered into it with a glowing handheld device. Always droll, I knew he was asking both as part of the usual chit-chat and as a way to begin his familiar "I can't stand working out" routine.

"Powerlifting, yes. Not bodybuilding." Most people don't know that bodybuilding, weightlifting, and powerlifting are different sports. Unless asked, I don't break down the differences; it's tiresome while simultaneously making me nervous that I'm being pedantic.

"Powerlifting. Bodybuilding. Really?! Still?" He didn't ask about the difference.

"Yup. I'm training myself and even coaching other people now, too."

"You are? That's great. I go to the gym. But I hate it. It's awful. Why do we do that to ourselves?" Without taking a breath, he launched into his usual tirade. "I mean, I know why we do it to ourselves. We have to. Well, you seem to like it. Do you have a trainer? I have a trainer and I go because I have to go. I mean, we all should go. But it makes me miserable. How did you get yourself to like it? I can tell, you love it! How do you love it?" he asked with sincerity, and I laughed, thinking it a rhetorical question.

"I'm serious! How can I learn to like it? I can't, can I? But I go," he continued.

"Oh!" I realized that he actually wanted me to answer him. "Well, you keep showing up, right? That's good. It's a process, I guess. I found something I loved. You've told me you love eyes and I know you love your work. You rarely take a vacation and you always seem to be happy to be working with your patients. You love doing this."

"I do. I love eyes." He paused, looked up, took a breath, and smiled a little wistfully before continuing the exam.

FINDING YOUR WORKOUT "WHY"

Americans seem resistant to admitting that it is normal to struggle with turning a new movement or wellness practice into a habit. This is never more apparent to me than when February rolls around, year after year. Every January 1, it seems like a large percentage of all the people I've ever met (and am friends with on Facebook) publicly resolve to make the upcoming year the year they start exercising regularly! And every January, the gym is busier than it is during the eleven other months, leaving me waiting for a squat rack and jockeying for twenty-pound dumbbells. But by February, I don't have to worry about crowds. According to the International Health Racquet and Sports Club Association, about eleven percent of gym memberships are sold in January, but by February, eighty percent of resolution-makers have fallen off the gym wagon.[1]

After my appointment, Dr. Friedman and I both went on to do the thing we loved: he saw more eyes, and I made my way to JDI Barbell to get some training in before coaching. It had been two and a half years since [   ]. I was still showing up and loving training, my back no longer gave me grief, and I had made progress with my PTSD. And in a surprising twist, I also found myself feeling more self-actualized than ever. I had become a National Academy of Sports

Medicine Certified Personal Trainer, deepened my trauma studies, begun to coach at JDI Barbell, and became the first trauma-informed strength coach I knew of.

"How did I get here?" I asked myself, replaying my interaction with the doctor and laughing at the sheer speed of his words. While some of the answers to that question were more obvious to me (seeking therapy, training, knowledge, support, wanting to be better for my family, and my own grit, among other things) I knew that the key was something else. How did I figure out what I needed, keep pursuing it, and find my joy in movement? How did I ever become someone who loved the gym, considering how much I used to hate it? Many of the other fitness professionals I know played team sports, or danced, or at least thought gym class and recess were fun when they were kids. I spent my middle school lunch and recess in the art room, and gym class silently praying not to be noticed. By high school, I wanted to have nothing to do with being in my body at all, let alone exercise. It was only under doctor's orders that I begrudgingly showed up at the gym when there seemed to be no other option for my pain. It took another three years for me to get comfortable enough with my strength to show up more willingly, which is where I eventually found my joy, along with transformative and healing relationships.

"But what about other people? Why did *they* show up?" I wondered to myself. With my clients, I can assess their individual reasons and really tailor a plan to their lifestyle. That's part of my job. But my micro-level understanding was highly specific to each individual and certainly couldn't be extrapolated to the general gym-goer. While I'd chat with some of my fellow lifters at JDI, I don't talk to lots of people in the gym for the most part, and certainly not at places like the YMCA (where I practiced my active recovery exercises). Other members and I would listen to our headphones and move in silence beside one another. I knew for myself, but I had no real sense as to why they kept showing up in spite of conditions of exhaustion, full schedules, other stressors, chronic pain, and more. I didn't know the details of their stories, but seeing them show up like I was reminded me they had stuff going on, too—at the end of the day, we're all only human. So, why did we keep at it when it felt so hard to do?

As someone who's made a 180-degree turn in their relationship with exercise, I feel like I'm in a unique position to help others start a new embodied movement practice, and one they're likely to keep. I want you to show up for yourself at the gym, fitness studio, playground, sidewalk, rock wall, or wherever you're motivated to do your movement practice.

Dr. Lisa Lewis is a counseling psychologist with a background in sports psychology, who also facilitates professional development for fitness professionals in areas where psychology meets physical wellness. I first met Lisa at a seminar in Boston, where she touched on one of her specialties: finding motivators to help clients maintain their fitness practice.

I told her a bit of my origin story, hoping she could help me pin down how I made the transition from gym class truant to exercise ambassador. And as the conversation unfolded, we identified a few truths around exercise.

Start Somewhere

First of all, you have to start your practice somewhere. In my case, I started because I had to, for the health of my back. Resentment aside, I showed up because the alternative—being in constant pain and having to spend countless hours lying down—seemed even worse.

Starting somewhere doesn't need to look like showing up to strength training under your doctor's orders. It could be trying out a spin class because you have a coupon, starting to walk because you'd like to participate in a charity walk in a few months' time, or getting on a bike because it's your best option for getting to work. Just by showing up for yourself in this way, even if you have to start a few times over, you are, as Lisa said to me, "giving yourself the opportunity to find what you like. And when you do, you're in!"

Relationships Heal

Lisa also reminded me of something I learned in my counseling program when she said the following: "One important thing I tell trainers all the time is that the relationship was the key to getting you in. Just like with counseling, no matter which orientation you like, the rapport with the client is what determines the outcome. And I would argue, though I don't have any data, that the same thing goes for the personal trainer relationship. That rapport is very pivotal."

This is the second truth about exercise we've established: relationships have the power to help us feel connected and even heal, even in the gym. There is growing interest in the role of good relationships, not just in counseling but in traditional healthcare and physical therapy, too.[2] A study of physical therapists treating chronic lower back pain (something familiar to many of us, as lower back pain has been identified as the leading cause of disability worldwide[3]) found that a therapeutic alliance, or solid relationship between the client and therapist, was associated with reduced pain for the client, and that positive interactions between the client and therapist "were associated with greater improvements in perceived effect of treatment, function, and reductions in pain and disability."[4]

Remember how Big Ed's presence made it okay for me to be in the gym despite my personal baggage? He'd created a safe space for me to show up and "get my reps in," as Lisa would say, and I found that it worked. I hated showing up at first, but being with Ed made the hour more enjoyable and I always felt better after moving.

Finding a healing relationship within the gym, like I did, feels amazing. But sometimes making more casual connections to others can be enough. Dr. Friedman shows up because he "has to." He didn't elaborate, but he's said he has a trainer and I happen to know he's been showing up to exercise for quite some time, despite hating it. Could there be something to their relationship that he appreciates, just maybe? I know that's the case with my husband, David. While he likes feeling healthy and vital, getting the opportunity to connect with George, his trainer, is fundamental in motivating him to show up and work out. I saw this play out during the early days of the COVID-19 pandemic, when gyms were shut down for quite some time in New York City. David had access to the home gym I built, but he skipped a few training days during this time—something that doesn't happen when he trains twice a week with George. "I miss George," he said to me one day, when I asked him if he was going to train at home. As we'll explore in the next chapter, feeling connected to others in the gym, yoga studio, or wherever you exercise, can help you feel grounded, safe, and regulated, which can be a motivator in itself.

Get Curious About Your Strengths

If you don't have access to a trainer, or someone who can create the place for you to start your movement practice, that doesn't mean you're a lost cause. Whether you work out alone by choice or due to limited access, this can be a good chance to deepen your relationship with yourself. "Be curious, look for what you are good at and find something you enjoy," Lisa said. "Maybe you are someone with excellent mobility who likes being bendy: start with yoga and run with it."

If you're naturally strong like me, maybe you'll get curious about strength training. Or perhaps you loved to dance as a child, which could be channeled into a barre, Zumba, or dance class at a local community center. If you really like the feeling of freedom that comes with moving quickly, ride a bike or run. Maybe you miss the monkey bars—playground-based workouts (I'm serious, these really exist!) might be made for you. Starting with your greatest loves and strengths creates the space to get curious, and even find other practices stemming from that.

Find Your Joy

During my conversation with Lisa, I realized I first became truly eager to work out when I began to practice Olympic weightlifting. I found so much joy in cultivating the new skills, developing strengths I already had, and working on the technique needed to lift heavy things up and over my head, that I would go out of my way to train. It took eight years of showing up, getting my reps in, and trying things like running, rowing, and yoga to stumble upon my joy: barbell sports.

Before I found it, I used to see vacations as a time to abandon everything on my chore list: paying bills, grocery shopping, cooking dinner, laundry, and working out. But once I found joy in barbell sports, I started incorporating workouts into our vacations; I'd do research in advance to find gyms to train in, and checking out barbell clubs in different cities and towns became part of the fun. I'll usually buy a day pass and a branded shirt if they're selling one, as a souvenir. On trips to places like Disney World, jam-packed with family activities, I'll set an alarm for 6:00 a.m. and get in a workout without cutting into the family's itinerary. There are always a couple of like-minded parents in the fitness centers having some "me time" before putting on Mickey Mouse ears and navigating the crowds and long lines in the Orlando heat. In fact, by taking time to ground through movement in the morning, I feel better facing the potentially over-stimulating Disney experience.

Finding motivation that comes from within us, making a wellness practice a habit, and ultimately finding the practices we love, is a process that asks us to start somewhere, be curious, and find our joy. Creating a sustainable practice is a process. If where you start doesn't immediately bring you joy, don't fret; remember you're *taking care* of yourself and sometimes things are more therapeutic than fun, and that's okay. Being curious will, over time, allow you to try different things and find your joy. In other words, just start with what you know and stay curious about what you don't.

TAKE ACTION
Get Curious About Your Strengths

Your strengths help you handle the stresses of life and engaging with your strengths also makes your life more fulfilling. Strengths aren't just things you're good at doing, but things you enjoy doing naturally and consistently. They are a good place to draw inspiration from if you want to embark on a new practice but don't know where to start. Focusing on your strengths is also useful for trauma work, since it gets you out of feeling stuck in a sense of weakness or pain and into a feeling of empowerment. In this exercise, you'll fill out the following form to help you identify a good place to start for creating your sustainable movement practice. Once you know your strengths, you can begin to figure out how to leverage them to lift whichever heavy things need moving in your life.

WHAT YOU WILL NEED:
A journal or a piece of paper
A writing instrument
A quiet, comfortable place to sit

DURATION:
20 minutes

Take a moment to feel yourself being supported by your cushion, chair, the floor, or wherever you're sitting. Really allow your weight to fall into the ground. Now begin by answering the questions below:

1. Out of everything you do in a given week, what do you enjoy doing the most?
2. Out of everything you've ever done, what did you enjoy the most?
3. What have you done in your life that came easiest to you, or felt the most natural?
4. Which tasks or practices do you consistently do now? Describe them.
5. What steps do you take to do them? What time or day of the week do you do them? What do you like about doing them?

Look at this list. Notice the traits, skills, and activities you have mentioned. These are some of your strengths—things you enjoy and do naturally, because you want to. With this list in hand, identify a kind of movement practice that you might associate with these traits, skills, or activities. Sometimes the translation is more obvious, such as enjoying listening to music or playing an instrument turning into a love of dance. Others are less obvious, but infinite connections are possible: perhaps you enjoy and excel in working collaboratively, which could translate to an intramural sport or group cross-training. Make sure to note whether any of your current practices are embodied, as you may find that certain tasks you already do demand a level of bodily awareness. Are any of these tasks empowering and do they increase your sense of agency?

As you contemplate these possibilities for movement, notice how you feel inside. Which activities spark a sense of curiosity and enjoyment? You'll probably have a more positive instant response to some ideas than others.

When you have identified one or more activities you feel open to trying, begin researching what you'll need to get started. You may also want to refer to your original intake form, which includes the conditions you'll need for your practice. And please remember, it's more than okay if you try something new and it doesn't work out for you. Stay curious, let it go, and try again.

CHAPTER TWELVE

Healing Your Relationships and Finding Connections

W E ARE ALL INTERCONNECTED. Our actions affect a larger ecosystem of people, places, and things outside of us. This is never clearer than when we experience trauma, as in this state, we often withdraw, act out, pick fights, or disappear—behaviors which ripple out to affect the people in our lives.

When you're healing from trauma, your behavior changes yet again. As we've explored in this book, healing gives you a stronger sense of your boundaries and allows you to more skillfully make your voice heard, trust yourself and others, and feel more empowered to act. Each change within you has an impact on your relations with others, so after you've started healing work, don't be surprised if you look around and realize your relationships are crying out for healing work, too. If you don't have many strong relationships, you may find yourself craving connection. Connecting with new people through support or interest groups, finding a therapist with whom you have a good rapport, and coming together with someone you care about for some relationship TLC, for example, can all be done at any point in your healing process. It need not wait until the end, for healing doesn't happen in a vacuum. You need others along the way—for motivation, as we saw in the last chapter, and for support.

After [   ] I felt like I had become a monster. Spending my days at the edges of my tolerance for stress, I was easily triggered and over- whelmed, which made me lash out in ways that felt like the darkest, meanest parts of me were coming to the surface. My outbursts could be triggered by anything that stressed my system: being overwhelmed by a loud sound, asked a favor, or presented with a change in plan, among other things. I also unwittingly set myself up for these crashes with constant training and limited recovery. I was pushing all my sys- tems to the limit and I never took the time to recover. The stress of trauma, and of overtraining fueled by unprocessed trauma, were leaving me with limited energetic resources to meet the inevitable stressors of life. I trained hard every day because the world didn't feel safe. I lost my connection to the most basic conditions I needed to live as a human.

I was full of spite and pushed hardest at the people I was closest to. I would yell at my loved ones, say hurtful things, or get up and leave the room or house for hours at a time. I knew I was just reacting to feeling overwhelmed, but I was afraid that I was morphing into someone else and would become malicious permanently. Everyone knew something was up, but it seemed no-one knew how to help—including me.

I felt certain my outbursts and disappearances were hurting my family, which in turn hurt me on top of what my trauma was doing. So, I pushed away from everyone, because no one felt truly safe. All of my relationships were tested, but none as much as mine and my husband's. No one would ever guess that looking at us now.

"You guys are like the ideal couple. I want to be in a relationship like yours," our twenty-something babysitter said when we returned from our weekly date night. David had probably said something sweet and cheesy to me before heading down the hall to check on our daugh- ter. David and I are a very secure and loving couple, and ours is a true nerd love story: in 2002, we met in a bookshop and the attraction was instantaneous. Over the next two decades, we grew together; both soft- ening over time, we now bring out each other's tenderness. Our mar- riage is a responsive and supple partnership. We don't just divide up the tasks—the division of labor is fluid, meeting both of us where we are at any given point so that we can truly support one another over the course of our lifetimes together. At the end of the day, we just really like each other and enjoy one another's company.

"Aw, yes. Thanks. Yeah, we are a pretty solid couple." I wasn't sure if my reply was good enough. This sweet young woman standing in front of me had big, round eyes and long, blond curls reminiscent of a Disney princess. Part of me felt compelled to gently share what I had learned over time: that solid relationships are not fairy tale romances. Fairy tales involve battles with dragons, trolls, and evil queens, and end "happily ever after" once the protagonists are united. The story of David and me was built through the unglamorous effort of hard work over the years since our meeting. I know we make it look easy now. Our sitter was one of many to say this to me. But the truth is that while we are a great match, we also fought to be here.

I didn't want her to think that David and I had some magic other people don't have. Instead, rather like a house, we had the raw materials for a good relationship, we built it, and we maintain it so that it continues to give us shelter and comfort. I continued, "Just so you know, it wasn't always easy and it took a lot of work. There was a time we didn't know if we were going to make it. That's actually where date night came from."

"Oh, wow," she said, her eyes growing even rounder, along with her mouth. "I'm glad you did. You guys are great."

LIFTING HEAVY THINGS IS NOT A SOLO SPORT

There was never a time in our relationship when David and I didn't argue. We moved in together after four months of dating, and shortly thereafter had an argument about whether his leaving socks in the living room was a sign of disrespect. (I said yes, he was disrespecting me with his socks, and he said he wasn't. I will yield now, eighteen years later, he was not.)

You can bet that after nearly two decades of living, eating, reading, and watching TV together, we've discovered things that irritate one another even more than socks. We are different people after all, with different habits and approaches to problems. Many of these annoyances are small: I manage to create (what seem to me) tiny pools of water in the bathroom and kitchen when I use the sink, and while I remain willfully blind to them, David inevitably grumbles when he leans against the counter or steps in a puddle in socked feet. He does the dishes nearly every night but often forgets to wash one pot or pan, and it will sit there until I inevitably need to scrub out the caked-on residue when I go to cook lunch the next day.

Other times, we do things that wear away at one another pretty quickly. David has a casual relationship to time and deadlines, whereas I'm pretty rigid about schedules. I struggle to take criticism, which means opening conversations with me about things I'm doing that bother him can feel potentially perilous for David.

But our differences, even the ones that produce conflict, are okay, because we know how to talk and work them out. First of all, we rarely address an issue in the moment of annoyance. Even letting just sixty seconds pass is a good idea. After a short pause, I might say, "Hey, I wanted to talk to you about scheduling. Can we do that now, or should we do it after dinner?" I start building the container for the conversation by creating a time for it. David might say to me, "Hey, I'm honestly asking because I'm hoping to find an easy solution—what were you doing when you created that puddle on the counter? And did you notice it?" He starts building the container by letting me know that he doesn't think I'm doing anything bad, he just wants to find a solution with me that works. Pausing, asking questions and listening to the answers, and respecting the other person's boundaries, all create the conditions to address the problem and move forward, just as they do in the gym.

We didn't come into our relationship knowing how to do this. Like everything else, we had to learn. We had a lot of it modeled for us in couples counseling.

If you haven't had constructive behavior modeled for you by your caregivers, friends, or mentors, you can't be expected to know how to react constructively in the best of circumstances. And if you are living with trauma it can feel a million times harder, because you may have to re-learn what it means to feel safe with your people. That's what happened to me. Before I could learn how to have constructive conversations around conflict, I had to learn to feel safe in the presence of others, including my husband.

About a year after I developed PTSD, we went into couples counseling and, over a few months, started to create a container in which I could feel safe in our marriage. We were honest in therapy and would then bring what we learned together to our respective private therapists as well. We also had homework, which we did, both separately and together. The biggest assignment was for us to have a weekly date night. For me, it was practice in trusting David to show up and help me feel safe out in the world. For David, it was practice in being there with me and emotional intimacy. Due to our sustained honesty, mutual hard work, and weekly ritual of date night, I began to feel safe again.

I know that engaging in these layers of therapy is unusual for many folks, but that's the kind of help David and I were comfortable with. Neither of us belongs to a faith that provides counsel, nor do we have people close to us that we could turn to about our marital strife. Therapy was the place where we could build on our resources together. We tended to what we had. We showed up each week until the two of us, and our therapist, agreed that we'd achieved our therapeutic goals. And to this day, we maintain date night as a source of joy that we happily look forward to each week.

One evening in 2015, shortly after we graduated from couples counseling, I turned to face him across the dining table and announced, "I'm pissed. I didn't know marriage would take so much work." Even though I was exhausted and meant what I said, I smiled as I said it. We had done enough work that a proclamation of this sort felt safe to say. In fact, being able to do so was an acknowledgment of how much hard work we had put in.

"Really? But that's what all the stories are about." David was genuinely surprised.

"No. No, they're not. Not the stories I know. The stories I know are about how hard it is to get together, not stay together. They all live happily ever after." I was thinking of books like *Pride and Prejudice*, fairy tales from childhood, and every rom-com I've ever watched. At the time, I had no idea what stories he was referring to. In retrospect, my response feels odd, as I don't read Jane Austen or believe in fairy tales. My favorite tales are coming-of-age stories and memoirs, which are all about resilience: about the people who helped the protagonist reach their destination, and others the protagonist might have lost along the way. In these stories, you see how interconnected we are and how what happens to us ripples out into our relationships. Sometimes the impact deepens the connection, as it did for David and me, but sometimes it severs it. That makes the stakes feel even higher.

I invite you to pause, check in, place one hand on your heart and one on your belly, and feel your weight being supported by the seat beneath you.

CONNECTION AS HEALING

Feeling connected to others is important to healing—in therapy, in the gym, and around the kitchen table. Remember, studies show that across all areas of healthcare, healing is found not only in the tools used, but in the relationship between the client and practitioner. From a body-based perspective, this is attributed to co-regulation, which is at the core of person-to-person connection. This is a psycho-biological phenomenon in which two nervous systems come together in a way necessary to feel safe. And you can't heal from trauma without feeling safe.

That said, when you have experienced being harmed by another person, co-regulation can feel dangerous. When you feel lonely but can't connect to others, your nervous system responds in the same way as when you're in danger; your cortisol level increases and you move into an activated state. Seeking out connection in this aroused condition doesn't have the healing effect we're looking for. Instead of conversation or deep listening, people may pick fights, act out, or engage in attention-seeking behavior. On the other hand, some people respond to the loneliness that comes from trauma by further withdrawing and isolating themselves.[1] In this situation you're in survival mode and your body doesn't understand that you actually have survived, that you are alive, so it continues to do what's necessary to protect itself.

If feeling safe is necessary to heal from trauma and co-regulation is required to feel safe, but you no longer have the ability to trust people, then you might find yourself in quite the bind. The good news is that you only need to start healing with one relationship. I found a therapist with whom I felt connected and safe. I trusted that she had the professional skills necessary to help me. Co-regulation can be found in any positive relationship where both parties show up in an authentic way, whether that's with a friend, co-worker, classmate, trainer, workout buddy, or even a pet. It's not limited to romantic relationships and therapists.

And these connections don't need to be related to your trauma story, either. Some places people find connections where one's trauma doesn't need to enter the picture are spiritual communities, dance studios, art classes, yoga studios, and gyms. I know people who have gotten sober with the support of the community they found in group cross-training gyms, and I know people who have found their closest confidante by asking for a spotting partner so they can feel safe when training a heavy bench press. As a coach, I've seen lifelong friendships formed, roommates found, and partnerships of all sorts established at the gym. Many of the same resources we use for embodied movement can be used to change and heal our relationships, too. And just as it took me time to settle into an embodied movement practice, I was able to eventually find that feeling with David, too. Trauma, in leaving us feeling disconnected from our loved ones, can rock even the strongest foundations.

That said, not all relationships can, or should, be mended. Not all of my friendships survived the aftermath of my trauma, which is not a bad thing. I shared my marriage not as a prescription for what you should do, but as an example of how trauma has a ripple effect on our relationships and networks.

Lifting heavy things together and trusting that your partner or teammates will allow you to push yourself and take risks, but help you out if you are in a jam, builds trust. I remember being in the free weights section, locking eyes with the only other woman there and smiling at each other, acknowledging the sisterhood of women who lift—a silent exchange that created a moment of grounding and sense of safety in a stimulating environment. It feels good to be seen and met with understanding.

If you picked up this book planning to train on your own, there are plenty of other places to find community outside of your movement practice. Classes of countless kinds and spiritual or worship groups are places you can look that aren't related to dealing with trauma. Ask yourself, what do you love? What have you wanted to learn how to do? Foreign language, dance, yoga, speechmaking, astrology, and Reiki classes are a few of the non-gym classes I've recommended to clients looking for community. And for something more explicitly therapeutic, there are support groups and group therapy of all kinds. I know people who rely on Alcoholics Anonymous for sustained support and connection, and those mending past harms through attending healing circles.

Recovery doesn't look like just going back to "normal" for any of your parts: when your muscles recover from strength training they don't just feel better, they physically change and get stronger. The same can be said about recovering from trauma. The fact is that the trauma happened. If you can integrate it into your story instead of having it dominate your narrative, including your relationships, you will make space to recover—not just to feel better, but stronger. David and I were rocked by trauma, but then we put in the work and we grew. We continue to grow. And in doing so, we're living more fulfilling lives both individually and together.

TAKE ACTION
Practice Co-Regulation

Deb Dana is a licensed clinical social worker who specializes in helping people explore and resolve the consequences of trauma safely. As she put it, "co-regulation is at the heart of positive relationships: work alliances, enduring friendships, intimate partnerships." She explains that it "creates a physiological platform of safety that supports a psychological story of security."[2] In other words, we become more centered in our window of tolerance when we find co-regulation, enabling us to feel safe.

Our nervous systems connect and find co-regulation through hearing the other person's tone of voice, seeing their facial expressions and body language, and feeling their touch. As we connect, our autonomic nervous systems sync up for a shared calming experience.

For this exercise you have two options. Option A is an exercise around helping you find someone to do healing work with, if that interests you. In the immediate aftermath of my trauma I didn't feel safe around anyone, and I had to find a therapist I felt I could trust enough to help me heal. It's hard to find counseling, coaching, or other resources when you're in crisis, but that's also when you need it most. Option B is an exercise to practice co-regulation with any consenting partner you already know. Ideally it should be done in person, but a video call works as well.

OPTION A

WHAT YOU WILL NEED:
A journal or a piece of paper
A writing instrument
Internet access

DURATION:
No set length of time

1. Starting with a blank piece of paper, create a list of what you are
    looking for in a practitioner. This may include:

    • Modality of choice (therapy, body work, energy work, fitness
      coaching, etc.)
    • Cost (fees, possible reduced rates, insurance coverage)
    • Area of focus (grief, eating disorder, substance abuse, sexual
      trauma, etc.)
    • Gender, age, race, and other preferred traits
    • Location

2. Once you have your list of conditions, start your search for the right
    practitioner online. The specifics of the search will vary based on
    what you're looking for, but a good place to start is by searching for
    professional associations related to a specific modality, which often
    have directories. You could also start by searching for resources for
    coping with whatever it is you're looking into.

3. As you search, make a note of any practitioners who fit some, or
    all, of your conditions. Geographic, financial, and other practical
    constraints will narrow your search, and you may need to cast a
    wider net.

4. Ideally, you'll find two or three practitioners who you think might
    be a good fit. Reach out to them and ask to schedule a consultation.
    Consultations usually last between fifteen minutes and an hour and
    are often done over the phone, or sometimes by video call or in
    person. They are also often free. This is an opportunity for you to get
    to know the practitioner a little bit and get a sense of what it would
    be like to work with them.

5. Before each consultation, take a few moments to ground yourself,
    feeling the surface beneath your feet and the seat supporting you.
    Check in with yourself and notice how you feel.

6. During each consultation be prepared to share why you are looking
    for their services, but don't forget to ask about how they work: their
    background, how often they meet with clients, their general sched-
    ule, and what their policies are. Listen mindfully to their answers,

checking in with yourself from time to time to see how you're feeling as the conversation progresses.

7. After each consultation, take another moment to notice how you feel.

8. Based on how well a practitioner meets your conditions and how you feel after the consultation, select the one you think will be the easiest for you to show up and work with.

OPTION B

WHAT YOU WILL NEED:

Someone you know, with whom you feel safe

Access to video calling if you can't see them in person

DURATION:

5 minutes

1. Before you start, while standing or seated, I encourage both of you to check in with yourselves. Take a moment to observe your body and how it feels using interoception. Are any sensations, images, impulses, or emotions surfacing? Notice them.

2. Find a connective position that you both feel comfortable in and can maintain throughout the exercise. This could be facing one another, where you're able to observe the other person's face and body language, or connecting through touch: holding hands, sitting back to back and leaning on one another, or hugging. If you can't be together physically, set up your video call so you can clearly see the other person's face and torso, at least.

3. Focus your attention on the connection you've established and notice what it's like to look at one other or be in physical contact together. Spend a minute or two here. Notice if your breathing is syncing up together and slowing down. Spend five or more cycles of breath together here.

4. I now invite you to check in with yourselves again. Observe your body and how it feels. What sensations, images, impulses, or emotions are surfacing now? Notice them.
5. Thank your partner and yourself for creating the space to practice co-regulation.

CHAPTER THIRTEEN

(Not) Telling Your Story

B EFORE YOU SHARE your own story, whether with an audience of one or of many, I encourage you to ask yourself the following questions:

> *Will it help me to share my story now with this person?*
> *Will it help this person?*
> *How will I feel afterwards?*
> *Will it harm me to tell my story?*
> *Will it harm someone else?*

By your story, I mean whatever personal narrative you're holding onto about your trauma. Perhaps it's the story of one very painful thing that happened to you, or maybe it's a series of small injuries that piled up over time, leaving you feeling diminished or ashamed. Maybe you're a private person or come from a culture that keeps personal information close to home, and what you're holding onto is something that just feels too personal to share. Your story doesn't have to be tremendous, riveting, or earth-shattering to be something you want to keep close to you.

I see a lot of people sharing their stories on social media these days. I do it, too. It is a natural medium for that—a tool that uses pictures, words, video and audio to foster connections and, potentially, greater

knowledge about healing trauma. Whenever I post, I try to do it
thoughtfully. I remember that what I share could trigger others dealing
with trauma or could leave me feeling vulnerable if people don't (or
do) engage with it. I try to read other people's posts mindfully as well,
because there are times when I've unwittingly stumbled onto someone's
unprocessed trauma story and it's left me feeling all kinds of awful:
flooded with painful feelings, triggered, worried about the person who
posted it, or a combination of all of these.

When I was writing this book, I kept all of this in mind. I didn't
share unprocessed trauma in these pages, nor even every trauma that I
have processed. I had boundaries for my own wellbeing and explained
them to you to inform your own.

One of the more triggering periods I had with Facebook was in
October 2017, after actress Alyssa Milano posted the tweet that made
#MeToo go viral. I was sitting at my dining table with my laptop open,
probably checking my email, writing a client program, or planning our
upcoming Halloween party, when without any conscious thought, my
finger typed an "f" in the address bar of my browser, which immediately
guessed "facebook.com." I had a habit of checking Facebook as a distrac-
tion. But the usual posts, like jokes, recipes, and baby photos, were few
and far between that day. My Facebook friends are almost all women or
gender non-conforming individuals I met through attending a women's
college and engaging in strength sports, and that day, nearly every post
in my feed was a wall of text describing an act of sexual violence committed against my friends, with the hashtag #MeToo at the end.

"What the . . ." I whispered to myself and scrolled, feeling an intense
amount of pain for my friends mixed with fear. "No, no, no, no, no,"
I muttered as I read one person's detailed account of a rape, which she'd
never shared before. I kept reading with dread, knowing that folks were
sharing unprocessed traumas very publicly and potentially being triggered. And all of that unprocessed pain was certainly triggering to me.
I became extremely dysregulated. Sliding down in my window of tolerance toward immobility, I crawled into bed and lay there unmoving,
wondering what the hell was going on.

The next day I googled #MeToo and learned about Alyssa Milano's tweet. For days I approached my social media feed with caution. It was dominated by stories of sexual violence and survivors looking for connection with others, but there was no one providing care, help, or explanations of what it can feel like when you disclose these stories. A year later, Pew Research found that #MeToo was used over nineteen million times on Twitter alone, and that personal stories were a key topic in tweets.[1]

I wanted to help every single person whose story I read but I didn't know what to do, and the pressure to share my own story felt real. I was torn. If I shared my story now, I knew I would feel like I was overriding my personal boundaries—something I had consciously decided I would no longer do. But I could feel my edges becoming brittle again. I wanted to be among my community. I wanted to help and be helped. As I was pulled between these two needs, safety and community, I could feel I was pressing against my edges.

It turns out I wasn't the only person sitting at home, reading stories and worrying about what to do. In 2019 I had the opportunity to hear Tarana Burke, founder of the Me Too Movement, speak at the International Trauma Conference. She had founded Just Be, a local grassroots organization uplifting black teen girls, in 2003, and in 2006 she began to use the words "me too" to raise awareness of sexual assault and abuse within the community. It was a way for vulnerable survivors participating in Just Be programs to find and express empathy without sharing their stories. They could just say "me too" and be part of the group healing.

She recounted her experience of learning about how #MeToo went viral after, unbeknownst to her, Alyssa Milano tweeted, "If you've been sexually harassed or assaulted write 'me too' as a reply to this tweet," inspiring thousands of comments, replies, retweets, and more original posts. Burke noted that Milano didn't know about her when she wrote her original post and passed the mic when Burke came forward to claim the movement.

Burke's friends alerted her to the trend on social media and she went to look. Seeing the movement spread before her eyes, she clicked on a random post. She read it and cried because "It was sad," she said. But like me, she was worried about what was now happening all over the world.

> *"I was concerned. There was all this spillage on the internet with no container to process. No guidance. Nobody saying, 'This is why you feel the way you feel.' Nobody saying, 'Once you disclose, you might experience this. Don't feel bad.'*
>
> *I think one of the greatest failings of that first week of #metoo going viral was with all the big national organizations that deal with sexual violence. I didn't see eight hundred numbers being pushed out. I didn't see PSAs. People should have jumped immediately on that and said, 'Listen, we haven't had a chance to talk about sexual violence nationally, #metoo has gone viral, we are experienced in this way, and this is how we can help you.' Everybody was a deer caught in the headlights."[2]*

Burke came forward with her small organization and five hundred Twitter followers (she now has 303,000) and began to organize this uncontained, emotional, painful movement. As she put it, "It was obvious people were looking for community."

After a few days I compromised. I wanted to be in a community, but I didn't feel compelled to share stories about my own experiences with sexual harassment and violence. I added my voice to the count and typed "#MeToo" into my Facebook post, and nothing else. I knew it would disappear into the deluge of other posts with the same hashtag like a drop into an overflowing bucket. But by using the phrase as Burke intended, just two words without a story, I found a safe way to be in this community.

I invite you to pause, check in,
and orient to your space.

SHARING IN A HEALTHY WAY

It isn't inherently damaging to share your story. As discussed in Chapter Twelve, we can heal from trauma through relationships. Finding someone to confide in and being met with support by them can be healing, whereas walking around with a secret can result in growing feelings of shame. In the last chapter, I touched on the healing power of connection through co-regulation. Connection also provides the opportunity to be met with empathy, which can be very empowering. That person to connect with will be different for everybody, whether it's a relative, a friend, a hotline worker, or a spiritual leader. Who you confide in is not as important as how they show up for you.

If you look at any modern screening tool for PTSD, there will be a question along these lines: "Do you feel distant or cut off from people?" Trauma often leaves survivors feeling alienated, but if you can tell your story to someone and are met with understanding and empathy, no matter the amount of rage, sadness, grief, or pain you've felt, you can begin to feel tethered to humanity again.

Unfortunately, not everyone will receive your story in a supportive way. My friend Rachel didn't respond well to mine, and she wasn't the only one. You might share your story and be met with blame— "You should have known better," or "What did you do to provoke them?" Perhaps you're met with toxic positivity, which is a kind of enforced positivity that doesn't allow space for the painful feelings ("Everything happens for a reason"), or maybe with disbelief ("Well, I've never seen them act like that"). Your audience might want to fix everything and give you a list of "shoulds." For sharing our story to be helpful, we need to be seen, heard, and held as we are.

Each of us gets to decide if we want to subject ourselves to that risk. As we explored in Chapter Nine, identifying your boundaries, feeling into and enforcing them, and recognizing their ability to change over time, is a big part of healing and thriving. Remember what happened when I sat at lunch with Rachel? Well, when I told my therapist about the incident, my muscles *didn't* tighten further, which told me it was safe to continue. My body knew that telling her would help me feel better, more grounded and less lonely. When confiding in someone, listen to your gut and your muscles. Are they holding on tight or are they hoping to let go? This is why we practice interoception, so that even under pressure we can go inside and hear what our body's telling us.

Although you may feel drawn to share your story with just a few people, you may also want to share your story widely. I've seen countless people who have come through a trauma driven to change the conditions that led to their trauma. Sometimes the change is small, like a shift in their personal priorities, and sometimes it's bigger, like creating a foundation or charity. Both are driven by wanting to change reality itself.

The desire to change one's circumstances for the better strikes me as entirely human. The world needs people who can do this to create gateways. Alyssa Milano helped push the Me Too Movement to the forefront of our societal awareness. When she and many other actresses came forward with allegations of sexual violence against the powerful Hollywood producer Harvey Weinstein, they didn't know whether they would be blacklisted from acting or not. But they did it anyway. We need people who can tolerate the doubters, victim blamers, naysayers, and extremists. They are the changemakers. In this case, they stopped Weinstein's abuse and set off a movement that rippled across the entertainment industry and into others.

Connection and the normalization of our traumatic experiences is something we crave as social creatures and as survivors. Survivor stories shared on large public platforms can normalize traumatic experiences for others who feel alone and ashamed. When Dr. Christine Blasey Ford testified against then-Supreme Court nominee Brett Kavanaugh, she brought the Me Too Movement into politics; Malala Yousafzai stood up to the Taliban in the name of education for girls; and in her memoir *Becoming*, First Lady Michelle Obama revealed that a lot of the good work she had done in her life went unrecognized because of the color of her skin, letting people know that despite her success she, too, has been deeply impacted by racism.

WHY NOT TO SHARE YOUR STORY

Sharing your story is not always safe. You may not be met with death threats, but you could be met with violence or harmful responses like judgment, dismissal, or disbelief. If the conditions of love and support from your immediate community aren't met, then you're nowhere near as likely to be resilient in the face of those who would challenge your story when shared.

Tarana Burke understood this in 2006 when she began to use "me too" as a quiet, safe way for marginalized women of color who had survived sexual violence to acknowledge to one another that they weren't alone. In seeing just two words, survivors' realities had been changed; maybe they weren't as estranged from their peers as they'd thought. They didn't need to share the whole story to find peace and connection, just the acknowledgment of seeing and being seen. Unlike many public figures in the movement, the women Burke was helping were sharing quietly in a way that ensured their safety, and were changing their reality from one of aloneness to one of feeling connected. They did so without their own public platforms, yet the platform they shared was big enough.

You might feel called to share your own story at some point, whether to feel a sense of community, to help someone else, or to find help for yourself. And it needn't be as public as social media. A friend or coworker could confide something in you and you might feel an impulse to share something personal, too. Someone might ask, "Why are you acting like that?" on an anniversary of a painful event. If you choose to see a trauma healing practitioner or therapist, you'll likely feel pulled to share your story with them. And the story in question, your "why," doesn't need to be something extraordinary-sounding. It may be about an accident, an arrest, an illness, divorce, job loss, or any number of other things, but whatever it was it overwhelmed you. Now you find it difficult to share, and when you're feeling pressured it's hard to know what to do. If you feel this way, sharing your story could ultimately leave you feeling more dysregulated. Remember, when we tell our trauma story before we have processed it, we time travel and feel the way we did back then.

But you don't have to tell your story. Even if they ask. Even if part of you wants to. Even if that is why you showed up that day. Consider this permission to choose not to disclose. Your story is yours to share. There is power in taking ownership of your story. Take your time with that feeling. I waited days before typing #MeToo into Facebook. In my private work with clients I rarely disclose more than I'd share publicly in my writing. I choose to share the lessons I've learned instead. Sharing my story has the power to help or to harm; sharing the lesson will at worst be neutral, and most likely help.

Like me, you can say as little or as much as you want to. Sharing your story isn't an all-or-nothing game. You can say, "Speaking from personal experience that I don't want to get into, I have found x, y, and z to be helpful." I've written a whole book sharing all sorts of stories and personal lessons in order to connect with, and hopefully help you, but I haven't said anything I did not want to share.

Finally, you're allowed to change your mind. While you cannot take back what's already been said, you can always stop part way through and say, "I'm going to stop here. I realize I don't feel comfortable continuing to share." And if you're met with pressure to keep going, you can say, "No." You can walk away. You don't have to respond.

This is the same sort of agency I talk about using in the gym: you have the right to say no to doing something during your workout that you don't want to do. In fact, this act can be quite empowering, which is also healing for many trauma survivors. You may feel like you're being rude or somehow violating some rules of social engagement, but your boundaries must be your priority and sharing when you aren't ready can leave you feeling very vulnerable and unsafe. Social conventions have a way of making us override our impulses to leave a conversation when we want to (among other things). I argue that honoring your boundaries, which are empowering and keep you safe, takes precedence over being polite, which often keeps us small.

If you can share your story from a place of resilience, one in which you feel confident that your audience's response will not level you and you will not overwhelm your audience, then by all means, consider going for it. It's your story to do with as you please. Public disclosure makes space for others who don't want to share their story but still want to feel seen and understood. But remember to also consider whether it will help you, as well as others.

USING EMBODIED PRACTICE FOR EMBODIED SHARING

Learning how and when to share your story has its roots in boundary work. Like working to heal relationships, knowing your boundaries is a learned skill. As discussed in Chapter Nine, trauma inherently damages our sense of boundaries and often makes it hard to stay with our bodies. Embodied movement helps us practice feeling those boundaries. Mindfully lifting heavy things teaches us how to recognize what's enough, before we get to too much. And training within a community can teach us who to trust and with what.

If you want to share your story to be of service to someone else, be certain to take the time to ground yourself first and check in with yourself as you speak, making sure to stay in the present. Go slow and start with just the headline. Then pause again. You can use the grounding tools provided in Chapter Four's Take Action or any other tool you find useful.

If a story is shared in a thoughtful, self-aware way, it can foster the connection we crave from one another. It can offer hope, too. On the other hand, if you're sharing your story when you haven't processed your experience and aren't ready to, you may find your body feels like it did back when the trauma happened: dysregulated and overwhelmed. And if you don't have the conditions in place to be resilient in the face of challenges to your story, sharing your story can be painful and possibly even compound your trauma.

I have found choosing to not share my story widely to be empowering. At first, I often chose not to share it because my brittle container made it feel unsafe. I suspected that in sharing I would feel too vulnerable and overwhelmed, and unable to function. After I began to repair my boundaries, feel safer in the world, and process my trauma, I realized that my story is mine and that I get to do what I want with it. That felt important and very good. I put a pin in that feeling and have come back to it since I started changing my reality, both by working with folks living with trauma and becoming a published writer of personal narrative pieces. I want to make it acceptable for people to feel okay about not sharing, too.

My story is mine to tell whomever I choose, whenever I choose. As it stands now, I have the option to ask myself those original questions: Will it help me to share my story now? Will it help this person? Will I feel better afterwards? I always have a choice and I check in with my body to figure out my answers. When I get a "yes," I know it's safe to share.

TAKE ACTION
Pause Before You Post

Navigating social media is a challenge to your nervous system in general, and more so if you have experienced trauma of any kind. If you aren't on social media, I will admit I'm a bit jealous of you. It's often seen as something that connects us. I know it allows me to see some of what's happening in the lives of old friends and relatives who I'm not in regular contact with. It's also integral to my professional network and has introduced me to a broader range of news outlets and forms of social activism. These are the great, useful aspects of social media.

But we also know that social media takes a heavy toll on its users. Existing studies have found links between social media usage and depression, anxiety, and loneliness.[3] And beyond studies, I know many people who take social media breaks because it makes them feel better. So while social media puts us in contact with one another, the connections we make there aren't the same as the healing connections we find when we can hear a person's voice, see their facial expressions and body language, and feel their touch.

I'm sharing this exercise in mindful posting with the full range of practical, useful, and harmful aspects of social media in mind. In it,

I invite you to observe how using social media affects your nervous system and to pause before sharing anything on social media, whether that's a repost or your own post, and examine your motivations and what the potential impact could be.

WHAT YOU WILL NEED:
The impulse to post something on social media
A device with internet connectivity

DURATION:
5 or more minutes

1. Schedule a time to check your social media feed. This can be the time you usually tend to check it.
2. Before you start, please take a moment to check in with yourself. Notice any sensations, images, impulses, emotions, or thoughts that surface as you anticipate checking social media.
3. When you feel ready, begin to engage with your feed. Pause periodically—every two or three scrolls—check in, and notice any changes to the sensations, images, impulses, emotions, or thoughts that you're having. If you forget to check in and just keep scrolling, notice that, too.
4. If you feel compelled to post something, repost, or "like" any content, I invite you to pause. Ask yourself:

    •   How do I feel right now?
    •   How big is that feeling?
    •   Am I sharing this because I'm overwhelmed with a big feeling and I want help holding it? If so, how can I ask for help with a big feeling in another way than reposting? Can I take this experience offline and find an in-person connection to help me regulate? If not, can I add my own words to this post to provide emotional context that might help foster connection with my social network?

- Will sharing this harm others? (In cases where potentially traumatic details are being reported, consider whether this is new information or you're repeating and amplifying a trauma story already known to your network.)
- Is there a way to share this information that will both help me and be mindful of others? (Hiding previews, content warnings, and summaries are all tools you can use to care for your network when sharing hard information.)

5. Check in again after you pause and notice any changes to the sensations, images, impulses, emotions, or thoughts that you're having.
6. If you still feel called to post or repost, consider anything that may have come up in your reflections.
7. After you post (or choose not to), check in with yourself one more time. Notice any changes following your action.
8. Lastly, when you're done looking at social media, step away from your device and do one final check-in. Notice any changes.

CHAPTER FOURTEEN

What Moves You?

H OW MANY TIMES have you started a new practice and promised yourself that this time, it was going to stick? I know I've done this again and again in my life. Creating a new practice that you stick with long enough for it to become part of your routine means creating change in your life. I want to help you make that change and create a practice that lasts. With this final chapter, I want to share some concrete tips to support you in fostering change in your life and seeking a movement practice that moves you, the way weightlifting moved me. Once you have that, sustaining your practice will become much easier.

Know Why You Are Showing Up

Whether you call it keeping your eye on the prize, pursuing your "why," or looking at the big picture, knowing why you've decided to do this very hard thing will help you to keep showing up for it. I show up to heal: to heal my back and my relationship with my body, to heal from trauma, and to heal in the face of the stressful things life throws my way.

Training doesn't only change the shape of my body, the chemicals it produces, and the density of my bones; it lifts my spirit and makes me feel expansive and empowered. It is for me a practice that alters both

171

my physiology and my spirit. I've sometimes jokingly said I was "off to church" when heading to the gym. Training is a ritual that I engage in to deepen my connections with myself and my community. I do it to process emotions, lift my spirit, and nourish something I still struggle to name, which is integral to the very essence of me.

And that's why I've kept showing up for myself, at least twice a week for years. Ask yourself what your reason is. Why did you pick up this book? Your path may share similarities to mine, but it will be different because your experience is unique to you, and it will reflect your own circumstances, lived experiences, strengths, joys, and interests.

Acknowledge and Accept That Creating a Practice Requires Change

No matter your "why," creating a practice that lasts means creating change. This might be a change in your schedule, your relationship to your body, your priorities, or some combination thereof. Whatever the change, it's helpful to acknowledge that you will benefit from it, even if you feel some ambivalence.

Conditions First

Remember Coach Kenny's cue to prepare for your practice with a solid setup. In this case, that setup involves doing some self-exploration and research, thoughtfully picking something you're likely to stick with, and putting the conditions in place to practice it. Many of the Take Action exercises in this book are intended to help you with just that. You're more likely to keep showing up if you've done the work of preparation beforehand. Identifying things you like to do, determining the conditions that need to be met for you to practice, and getting equipment to help make this practice more efficient are forms of preparation that'll make showing up easier. Cover these bases and it's more likely that you'll keep showing up until it's become so woven into your schedule that it's just another habit.

Remember That Creating a Practice Is a Process

You don't just wake up one day and have a practice. It is a process. But the good news is that if you've picked up this book and read this far, you're already in the process! Congratulations. Even if you haven't done the exercises or given practical thought to what an embodied movement practice would look like for you, you've become aware that it's possible and what it might look and feel like generally. It can be difficult to move on from this point, and if you're feeling stuck, ask yourself why.

For a long time, I didn't think I could run around, lift more than I weigh, or even be friends with my body. Maybe as you're reading this you don't exactly feel unable to start something new, but you're thinking, "Why bother?" because you don't feel like you can make a practice stick. You may even be looking at the exercise equipment collecting dust in the corner of your basement, or at the twice-used gym membership card sitting in your wallet, as proof of your perceived inability. Maybe your memories of being picked last in gym class make you want to never move your body again, or maybe you've tried to get going in the past but couldn't reach your goals.

I have experienced every single one of these hypothetical scenarios. I hear you. However, once I let myself imagine what it would be like to spend my days in less pain, the idea of that was enough to motivate me to start the process of changing my life.

I can urge you to try again and try it differently until I'm blue in the face, but sometimes what we need is a life event to shake things up and spur us on toward action. You may be waiting for such a thing to happen. In the meantime, know that you are truly deserving of this effort whenever the time is right to make it. Although it might be hard, you *are* capable of finding your joyful movement and cultivating an embodied movement practice.

Some of you are already deep in the process of creating your practice: doing the exercises in this book, researching options for yourself, or ordering the equipment you need to start. Whether you're doing these things willingly or begrudgingly, you are putting the conditions in place to create your practice. The Take Action exercises throughout this book will help you identify your resources, goals, and strengths, and ask you to meditate on the conditions you need for healing. You are learning how to cue yourself to make your practice embodied and how to use arousal and recovery to create a more resilient nervous system. You're getting prepared. If you haven't set yourself a start date, do so now. And if your activity depends on good weather, set a rain date or two. Make a promise to yourself that you're going to start on that date. If you have someone supportive in your life, let them know how they can help hold you accountable to showing up—maybe they can call you on the day or drive you to your workout.

Show Up for Yourself

Show up. Because once you show up to practice, no matter how you do it, you're doing the thing—you are practicing! Let's acknowledge that that's a big deal. You are implementing the plan you created for yourself. Now it's important for you to support your effort in a way that keeps you showing up. You'll find it helpful to have some of the following things in place:

- **Social support,** like a workout buddy or a supportive friend who likes to hear about your small successes, can be really helpful. This is a positive way to feel a sense of accountability. When I trained with Ed, he would celebrate my small victories in the gym. I'd also share every new bit of progress with David, describing the movements every evening after I trained. Having him bear witness to my successes created space for me to get excited for myself.

- **Have realistic expectations** for yourself. Expect to improve but also expect to struggle with some new things and possibly not like every moment. Be prepared to have days where you become dysregulated or overwhelmed. Know that you have the tools to get regulated and grounded when you need to, through either visual or auditory orienting (page 63) and cool down practices (page 132).

- **Be flexible and willing to change course.** Understand that at some point you might have to take time off when illness or other life circumstances render you unable to practice for days, or even weeks. That is okay. All your progress will not be lost and can easily be regained when you return. I've had clients who had to take time off for injury and worried that in doing so, everything they worked for would disappear. This has never been the case. If you've been building a practice for two months and then have to take three weeks off due to a flu, you haven't lost everything you gained in those two months of work. You might experience a bit of a setback, but it generally won't take even three weeks to get back to where you were.
- **Celebrate your growth.** Have a way to measure every small bit of progress you make, so that when you feel like you aren't making any because the changes so far aren't sea changes, you can look at your record of achievements. I track all of my clients' work: every day, every exercise, every rep, and every weight lifted. I also ask them about their day and invite them to notice when they did something important outside of the gym, like using their agency or practicing an act of self-care. Just like sharing small successes with a loved one, this too creates the opportunity to observe incremental progress as it happens.
- **Have clear goals** so you can remind yourself why you're doing this. In the Take Action in Chapter One, I asked you to come up with reasons for your embodied movement practice. Your reasons are the foundation of your goals. The difference between the two is that goals are specific, measurable, achievable, and time-bound expressions of your reason. For example, if your reason is to mitigate back pain, the goal might be to go a week pain-free, then a month, and so on. Reasons are why you picked up this book and have come this far in reading it. When you're starting something new, it can be helpful to regularly remind yourself why you're doing things and to demonstrate that what you're doing is getting you closer to your goals. When the going gets tough, I sometimes write my goals on my bathroom mirror with a dry erase marker to remind myself why

I ought to keep showing up. It's easy to lose sight of the big picture when you're going through a rough patch. Staying with an action for a prolonged period is hard and you'll benefit from lots of support. As an aside, I think it's important to note that I have had goals I never met, and they were just as important as the goals I did meet because they got me to keep showing up. For example, I had two competition-related goals I never met: competing in Olympic weightlifting and qualifying for nationals in powerlifting. I worked toward those goals and when I realized that training to compete wasn't serving me anymore, I set different goals that were more aligned with my reasons for training.

If you're regularly carving out time and showing up to practice embodied movement, then you have a regular embodied movement practice. Perhaps you go to the gym and lift weights twice a week, run every other morning, attend Zumba class three nights a week, practice yoga with a recording before bed every night, or ride your Peloton during your lunch break. You're showing up and doing the thing you planned to do, and using the tools you learned in this book to make it mindful and therapeutic.

If this is you, pause and acknowledge the feeling of having achieved what you set out to do! I hope you've taken time to celebrate this big accomplishment. If you aren't there yet, I encourage you to take a moment now to imagine what it might feel like to reach that point, and remind yourself why you're putting the work in. I had a client who was very driven and a high-performing achiever. She was a young mother, a lawyer, and a powerlifter. She worked so hard to find a way to show up and train three times a week, no matter her schedule. But sometimes she couldn't quite make it for all three, because life happens.

"I wasn't able to do three times a week for week two and three because the baby and my husband were sick and I have a big case. And I feel so bad about it," she once said.

"You showed up twice. You trained. You recorded yourself and sent me videos to review. Remember you are doing so much else besides this.

You have work, and home, and a whole life you are living. You are showing up and practicing when it works for you. This practice, training, is about taking care of you. That's what you did this month. That is awesome!"

"Yeah, you're right," she hesitantly agreed, like she suspected I might be right but wasn't sure yet.

"Yes, I know I am right," I said with a small smile.

"Yeah, you're right," she affirmed with more certainty. "I am showing up for myself in lots of ways and that's big." Her smile met mine and her face brightened. She knew it and felt it to be true. Over the years she has continued to train, taking breaks when needed. She always comes back to strength training. Initially she thought a regular practice meant she was going to train hard three times a week, come hell or high water. But learning to honor her body was part of the practice, whether that meant training or taking a break for her overall health and well-being. Practices you do for your own wellness need to be holistic and account for all the other parts of your life. Sometimes you need rest and sometimes you need to tend to other things. Once she learned that, her practice became more sustainable for the long haul.

If you have found that you struggle sustaining your practice, ask yourself: are you looking at the practice holistically and within the context of your whole life? Are you meeting the conditions you laid out, and are your goals realistic? Revisiting these things and accounting for them in your plan will allow you to plan for sustainability.

Maybe you are not a planner and are more impulsive. I often throw myself into things blind, only later to say, "oops." I'm working at being okay with discovering that I'm really terrible at certain things, and knowing that (a) I can recover and (b) it's not a reflection of my own worth if I had a bad experience with a new activity. Without that outlook it can be really easy to be levelled by lack of planning. Give some thought to what *you* need to help you get back on the proverbial horse by revisiting your conditions from the Take Action in Chapter One and take the steps necessary to put those conditions in place.

*I invite you to pause, check in, and sit with the notion that
you have already begun to create your practice by reading this
book. Perhaps you can note how it feels to acknowledge this.*

Even if you start your practice begrudgingly, like I did, if you begin
to really tune in to how good it feels to achieve a small success and get
better at doing stuff you once thought you couldn't do, it will get easier
to show up. Next thing you know you may be showing up willingly,
even joyfully! To this day those small successes are why I keep showing
up again and again, along with the regulation, grounding, and emotional processing I gain from lifting heavy things. I believe the same
will be true for you. If you continue to celebrate small victories, stay
curious about your body and how it moves, and learn to be gentle with
yourself; if you can accept that you (and everyone else who is engaging
in a movement practice) are going to be confronted with things that are
hard to do, that you are going to make mistakes and have setbacks, that
you are going to have bad days, and that all of this is normal, you will
find yourself with a regular practice.

I wrote this book so that you would feel equipped to turn any
movement practice that calls to you into an embodied and sustainable
regular practice. It is my hope that you do so, and that along the way
you will find great joy and discover what moves you. I know that if you
stick with your practice in all its forms you will create conditions to not
only help you heal from trauma but begin to thrive. Cultivating a relationship with your whole self—not just your thoughts, or your feelings,
or your spirit in silos, but together as one—is empowering and energiz-
ing. I believe it can do for you what it has done for me and many of my
clients: foster a greater understanding and appreciation of yourself, help
you feel better, and empower you to lift your heavy things.

TAKE ACTION
Pause Before You Move

When I work with clients it is always my intent to render myself unnecessary. I consider it a success when a client feels equipped to move on from our work together and begin practicing without my support. I see myself as the woman at reception orienting you to the practice and showing you some of your resources, but this is your practice for you to cultivate. You are an expert in yourself and you're the agent that is creating your practice. So rather than always turning to me, I want folks to turn to themselves and ask, "What do I need today?"

This exercise can be done whenever you are feeling uncertain of what you need in a given moment, but I always do it before I practice, and I ask the same of my clients. It is the beginning of a conversation with the self that gets you to where you are in this very moment.

Before you practice, no matter the emotions and energy you are bringing with you that day, I invite you to pause, check in with yourself, and ask, "What do I need today?" I then encourage you to honor that.

WHAT YOU WILL NEED:
Yourself

DURATION:
5 minutes

1. Take a moment to situate yourself in a place where you feel safe to turn inwards. You can do this at home, or in your car or a changing room if you are practicing outside your home.
2. Start by grounding. With your eyes open or closed feel the ground beneath your seat and your feet. Next I invite you to check in with yourself and see what if anything grabs your attention. This could be a sensation, thought, or feeling. You might notice something like a flutter in your belly or tension in your back. Maybe you feel nervous or excited. Maybe you are thinking about what you are going to have for lunch today. You don't need to do anything with

whatever comes up, just note it. It is information about how you feel or what's on your mind at this present moment before you get moving.

3. Ask yourself, "What do I need today?" Again, what arises might be a sensation, thought, or feeling. You may find that initial thing that came up wants your attention. Maybe you need to tend to the tension in your body while you move, move in a way that lets you shake off excess arousal, or maybe you need a snack before you get to it.

4. Take another moment or two to feel the ground again. When you are ready to, I invite you to orient to the space around you by identifying three blue things, three red things, and three yellow things, or by listening first to sounds near and then to sounds farther and farther away, then coming back to the space you are in.

5. From here, try to honor whatever it was that your body said it needed as you move into your practice. That might mean making a change or two to the day's program; usually in the warm-up; seldom does it mean a complete overhaul, in my experience. Learning how to adjust your practice while still honoring the goals you have for it is part of the practice as well.

RESOURCE GUIDE

I AM OFTEN ASKED FOR reading lists and referrals and I thought this might be helpful to you too. What follows is a list of resources that I have used personally, and that have informed the practices I share in this book. That said, not all of the titles, classes, or practitioners will be for you. No one is for everyone; not me and not any other teacher or practitioner out there. Consider this list a series of possibilities for next steps. Please continue to use the Take Action exercises in this book to help you be discerning and stay in conversation with your whole self as you choose what to read and who to work with as you move ahead on your path.

BOOKS

The Body Keeps the Score: Brain, Mind, and Body in the Healing of Trauma
BY BESSEL VAN DER KOLK

Reading this book was a major turning point in my life. This is the book that gave me hope when I had so little, and confirmed my suspicion that my back problems were inextricably linked to my PTSD. Bessel van der Kolk, a clinician, researcher, and teacher, has contributed tremendously to the field of trauma study. *The Body Keeps the Score* explores how trauma literally changes the brain and the body and presents a number of promising body-based treatments for trauma, explaining not just what each treatment is but why it works. A word of caution: this is a challenging read that many people—with trauma and without—may find triggering.

Overcoming Trauma Through Yoga AND
Trauma Sensitive Yoga—Bringing the Body into Treatment
BY DAVID EMERSON

David Emerson is the founder of Trauma Center Trauma Sensitive Yoga (TCTSY) for the Justice Resource Institute in Massachusetts, an evidence-based practice for healing psychological trauma. Both titles explain not just TCTSY forms but also the rationale behind the practice, which has many parallels to the trauma-sensitive approach I employ with my clients.

Waking the Tiger AND
In an Unspoken Voice
BY PETER LEVINE

Peter Levine, the creator of Somatic Experiencing, is a psychologist with a background in biophysics. He has spent more than forty years studying stress. Both titles explain his findings in biology, neuroscience, and body-oriented psychotherapy, and provide a framework for understanding and working with trauma through the body. *Waking the Tiger* guides the reader through the process. *In an Unspoken Voice* is more of an academic book.

The Polyvagal Theory in Therapy: Engaging the Rhythm of Regulation
BY DEB DANA

Deb Dana is a Licensed Clinical Social Worker who specializes in using trauma work and has worked closely with Stephen Porges, the creator of polyvagal theory. This book clearly explains polyvagal theory, why it is important when working with trauma, and how to apply this theory in practice. It is intended for clinicians who want to understand and integrate polyvagal theory into their practice and I found it helpful for my own practice specializing in working with trauma.

The authors featured here also teach professional trainings. If you are interested in experiential learning, I recommend checking them out.

ORGANIZATIONS FOR FURTHER STUDY OF MOVEMENT FOR TRAUMA BEYOND YOGA

Trauma-Informed Weight Lifting

Based in Minneapolis, these workshops are for trainers and coaches. They combine lecture, demonstration, and case studies for hands-on applied learning.

TRAUMAINFORMEDWEIGHTLIFTING.COM

DIRECTORIES OF TRAUMA-SENSITIVE MOVEMENT PRACTITIONERS, BODYWORKERS, AND SOMATIC EXPERIENCING PRACTITIONERS

Movement@Home

LAURAKHOUDARI.COM

Following stay at home orders in the spring of 2020, I created a crowd-sourced directory of trauma-sensitive and Health at Every Size–aligned movement practitioners offering remote at-home services. These practitioners vary in specialty, modality, and cost.

The Breathe Network

THEBREATHENETWORK.ORG

The Breathe Network connects survivors of sexual violence with healing arts practitioners that offer sliding-scale, trauma-informed, holistic support. They also provide education and training for professionals in best practices for delivering survivor-centered, trauma-informed care.

Somatic Experiencing Trauma Institute Practitioner Directory

DIRECTORY.TRAUMAHEALING.ORG

The Somatic Experiencing Trauma Institute offers a global directory of Somatic Experiencing Practitioners. Practitioners vary in modality and specialty.

ACKNOWLEDGMENTS

WRITING AND PUBLISHING A BOOK takes a village, and I will be forever grateful to the community of bright, supportive, honest, and compassionate people who helped me write mine.

Let me start by thanking the folks who helped me get from my moment of epiphany—"I have a book in me!"—to being an author and holding a copy of my own book. Thank you to my literary coach, book doula, and guide through the land of all things biblio, Lisa Weinert. Thank you to my editor, Jennifer Kurdyla, who has patiently and kindly helped me become a better writer over the last year and a half and to my copy editor, Sydney Radclyffe, who helped make sure there was clarity throughout this book. And thank you to my publisher, Maggie Langrick at LifeTree Media, for believing in this project from early in its inception. I am grateful for how you and your team worked tirelessly to make sure that this book, and its message, would be read far and wide.

I would be remiss if I did not thank the big players in my healing journey. Thank you, Ed Williams, for helping me heal my body and making the space for me to feel okay as I discovered my love of strength training. And thank you to my therapist, who helped me heal my spirit and my relationships when I was afraid they were beyond repair. Thank you to Trevor Rappa for being the understanding physical therapist I needed, and thank you to my coaches, Jesse Irizarry and Kenny Bretania, for giving me a place to safely lift heavy things and be with my joy.

I will always be grateful to my teachers, Maureen Gallagher, Dave Berger, and Jane Clapp, and to all of those who have taught me through their own books. Thank you for enriching my path as a practitioner and teacher. Thank you to my clients for teaching me, too. I learn so much from working with each and every one of you.

And to my friends and family, I feel as if there are no words grand enough to express my gratitude, so hopefully this—combined with some delicious home-cooked meals—will do. Thank you to Crystal Alberts for giving me hours of feedback on my writing in college and for supporting me as I navigated the whole making-a-book process. Thank you to Kate DeBow, Wendy Fisher, and Martine Audet for cheering me on regularly via text and phone. Thank you to all of you who read passages, tried out exercises, and got excited for me. Thank you to my mother, a writer in her own right, for helping me become a writer, too; and to my father for supporting this craft. Thank you to my aunt Nancy and uncle Michael for frequently reminding me that writing this book is a huge accomplishment. Thank you to Cathy, Charlie, and Heather for letting me know how proud you are of me. And most of all, thank you to my biggest champions and daily supporters, David and Gloria. I seriously could not have done this without you. You are my most favorite people in the world and I love you more than any acknowledgment could ever capture.

ENDNOTES

CHAPTER ONE

1   Judith Herman, *Trauma and Recovery: The Aftermath of Violence—From Domestic Abuse to Political Terror* (New York: Basic Books, 1992), 160.

2   Paul D. Loprinzi, Jeremy P. Loenneke, "Engagement in Muscular Strengthening Activities is Associated with Better Sleep," *Preventive Medicine Reports* 2 (2015): 927–929.

3   Erika N. Smith-Marek, Joyce Baptist, Chandra Lasley, and Jessica D. Cless, "'I Don't Like Being That Hyperaware of My Body': Women Survivors of Sexual Violence and Their Experience of Exercise," *Qualitative Health Research* 28, no. 1 (2018).

CHAPTER TWO

1   John LaRosa, "$71 Billion U.S. Weight Loss Industry Pivots to Survive Pandemic," MarketResearch.com, June 3, 2020, blog.marketresearch.com /71-billion-u.s.-weight-loss-market-pivots-to-survive-pandemic.

2   S. M. Phelan, D. J. Burgess, M. W. Yeazel, et al., "Impact of Weight Bias and Stigma on Quality of Care and Outcomes for Patients with Obesity," *Obesity Reviews: an Official Journal of the International Association for the Study of Obesity* 16, no. 4: 319–326.

3   National Eating Disorders Association, "What Are Eating Disorders" (PDF), 2012, nationaleatingdisorders.org/sites/default/files /ResourceHandouts/GeneralStatistics.pdf.

4   Matt McGorry, "My Journey Toward Radical Body Positivity," Human Parts (Medium), May 22, 2020, humanparts.medium.com/my-journey-toward -radical-body-positivity-3412796df8ff.

CHAPTER SIX

1   Somatic Experiencing Trauma Institute, "What is Somatic Experiencing®?" traumahealing.org/about-us.

2   Somatic Experiencing Trauma Institute, "Somatic Experiencing® -- Ray's Story," YouTube video, February 28, 2014, youtube.com/watch?v =bjeJC86RBgE.

CHAPTER SEVEN

1   Laura Schmalzal, Mardi A. Crane-Godreu, and Peter Payne, "Movement-Based Embodied Contemplative Practices: Definitions and Paradigms," *Frontiers in Human Neuroscience* 8, no. 205 (2014).

2   The Good Body, "Yoga Statistics," accessed September 25, 2020, thegoodbody.com/yoga-statistics.

3   Ted Alcorn, "Is This the End of the New York Yoga Studio," *The New York Times*, September 17, 2020, nyti.ms/3c5nFd7.

CHAPTER EIGHT

1   Judith Herman, *Trauma and Recovery: The Aftermath of Violence—From Domestic Abuse to Political Terror* (New York: Basic Books, 1992), 133.

CHAPTER NINE

1   Alexandra Black Larcom, "5 Things That Will Help Your Gym Members Stick with Their Exercise Habits," IHRSA, December 23, 2019, ihrsa.org/improve-your-club/5-things-that-will-help-your-gym-members -stick-to-their-exercise-habits.

2   Rafael Zambelli Pinto, Manuela L. Ferreira, Vinicius C. Oliveia, et al., "Patient-Centered Communication is Associated with Positive Therapeutic Alliance: a Systematic Review," *Journal of Physiotherapy* 58, no. 2 (2012): 77–87.

3   Jan Hartvigsen, Mark J. Hancock, Alice Kongsted, et al., "What Low Back Pain is and Why We Need to Pay Attention," *Lancet* 391, no. 10137 (2018): 2356–2367.

4   Paulo H. Ferreira, Manuela L. Ferreira, Christopher G. Maher, et al., "The Therapeutic Alliance Between Clinicians and Patients Predicts Outcome in Chronic Low Back Pain," *Physical Therapy* 93, no. 4 (2013): 470–478.

CHAPTER TWELVE

1   Deb Dana, *The Polyvagal Theory in Therapy: Engaging the Rhythm of Regulation* (New York: W.W. Norton, 2018), 44–46.

2   Dana, *The Polyvagal Theory in Therapy*, 44–46.

CHAPTER THIRTEEN

1   Monica Anderson and Skye Toor, "How Social Media Users Have
     Discussed Sexual Harassment Since #metoo Went Viral," Pew Research
     Center, October 11, 2018. pewresearch.org/fact-tank/2018/10/11/how
     -social-media-users-have-discussed-sexual-harassment-since-metoo-went
     -viral.

2   Tarana Burke and Licia Sky, "Me Too: At the Intersection of Sexual
     Violence and Racial Justice—A Fireside Chat with Tarana Burke," 30th
     Annual International Trauma Conference, Trauma Research Foundation,
     Boston, May 31, 2019.

3   Phil Reed, "Anxiety and Social Media Use," *Psychology Today*,
     February 3, 2020, psychologytoday.com/us/blog/digital-world-real
     -world/202002/anxiety-and-social-media-use.

INDEX

ABOUT THE AUTHOR

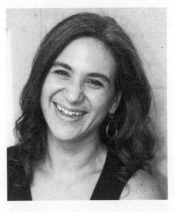

Laura Khoudari is a trauma practitioner, certified personal trainer, and corrective exercise specialist. She lives in New York City with her husband, daughter, and their two cats.

Learn more about her work and offerings at laurakhoudari.com.